CONGENITAL HEART DISEASE IN ADOLESCENTS AND ADULTS

Developments in Cardiovascular Medicine

VOLUME 136

Congenital heart disease in adolescents and adults

Edited by

JOHN HESS, MD, PhD

Professor of Pediatric Cardiology,
Sophia Children's Hospital,
Rotterdam, The Netherlands

and

GEORGE R. SUTHERLAND, MD

Consultant Cardiologist,
Western General Hospital,
Edinburgh, UK

Kluwer Academic Publishers

DORDRECHT / BOSTON / LONDON

Library of Congress Cataloging-in-Publication Data

Congenital heart disease in adolescents and adults / edited by John
  Hess and George R. Sutherland.
      p.   cm. -- (Developments in cardiovascular medicine ; v. 136)
   Includes index.
   ISBN 0-7923-1862-5 (HB : alk. paper)
   1. Congenital heart disease--Congresses. 2. Congenital heart
 disease in adolescence--Congresses.   I. Hess, John.
 II. Sutherland, George R.   III. Series.
   [DNLM: 1. Heart Defects, Congenital--congresses.   W1 DE997VME v.
 136 / WG 220 C74955]
 RC687.C664   1993
 616.1'2043--dc20
 DNLM/DLC
 for Library of Congress   92-49625

ISBN 0-7923-1862-5

Published by Kluwer Academic Publishers,
P.O. Box 17, 3300 AA Dordrecht, The Netherlands.

Kluwer Academic Publishers incorporates
the publishing programmes of
D. Reidel, Martinus Nijhoff, Dr W. Junk and MTP Press.

Sold and distributed in the U.S.A. and Canada
by Kluwer Academic Publishers,
101 Philip Drive, Norwell, MA 02061, U.S.A.

In all other countries, sold and distributed
by Kluwer Academic Publishers Group,
P.O. Box 322, 3300 AH Dordrecht, The Netherlands.

Printed on acid-free paper

Contents

List of contributors

EDWARD J. BAKER
  Department of Paediatric Cardiology, Guy's Hospital, St. Thomas Street, London SE1 9RT, UK

MARGREET TH.E. BINK-BOELKENS
  Department of Pediatrics, University Hospital Groningen, Oostersingel 59, 9713 EZ Groningen, The Netherlands

A.J.J.C. BOGERS
  Department of Thoracic Surgery, Dijkzigt Hospital, P.O. Box 1738, 3000 DR Rotterdam, The Netherlands
  Co-author Chapter 14: B. Mochtar

JACOB DANKERT
  Department of Medical Microbiology, University Hospital Amsterdam, Meibergdreef 15, 1105 AZ Amsterdam, The Netherlands

NYNKE J. ELZENGA
  Department of Pediatrics, University Hospital Groningen, Oostersingel 59, 9713 EZ Groningen, The Netherlands

ARTHUR GARSON JR.
  Pediatric Cardiology, Texas Children's Hospital, 6621 Fannin, Houston, TX 77030, USA

LIV HATLE
  Cardiology Division, University of Trondheim Medical School, Region-sykehuset, N-7006 Trondheim, Norway
  Presently at: Department of Cardiovascular Diseases, King Faisal Specialist Hospital, P.O. Box 3354, Riyadh, Saudi-Arabia.

JOHN HESS
  Department of Pediatric Cardiology, Sophia Children's Hospital, Gordelweg 160, 3038 GE Rotterdam, The Netherlands

FREDERIK K. LOTGERING
  Department of Gynaecology & Obstetrics, EE2283, Dijkzigt Hospital, P.O. Box 1738, 3000 DR Rotterdam, The Netherlands

DOUGLAS D. MAIR
  Department of Pediatric Cardiology, Mayo Clinic, Rochester, MN 55905, USA

JANE SOMERVILLE
  Grown-up Congenital Heart Unit, Royal Brompton and National Heart Hospital, Sydney Street, London SW3 6NP, UK

GEORGE R. SUTHERLAND
  Consultant Cardiologist, Western General Hospital, Crewe Road, Edinburgh EH4 2XU, UK
  Co-author: Oliver F.W. Stümper

ELISABETH M.W.J. UTENS
  Department of Medical Psychology and Psychotherapy, Erasmus University, P.O. Box 1738, 3000 DR Rotterdam, The Netherlands
  Co-author: Rudolph A.M. Erdman

C.A. WAGENVOORT
  Department of P.A. I, Erasmus University, P.O. Box 1738, 3000 DR Rotterdam, The Netherlands

MAARTEN WITSENBURG
  Department of Paediatrics, Sophia Children's Hospital, Gordelweg 160, 3038 GE Rotterdam, The Netherlands

Preface

In May 1990, the First International Symposium on Congenital Heart Disease in Adolescents and Adults was organized in Rotterdam. During these three days' Symposium an overview of the many new problems facing the adult and pediatric cardiologist as well as the cardiac surgeon in this rapidly increasing subgroup of the adolescent and adult cardiac population was given. Challenges, controversies, uncertainties and questions were presented and discussed with great enthusiasm.

We are greatful that most speakers who participated in this symposium, were willing to write a chapter on their presented topics to be edited in book-form.

The final result is here. We hope, it will be of value for both to the adult and pediatric cardiologist and other colleagues, who have to undertake the care of this group of patients, whose management poses such unique problems.

J.H.
G.S.

1. The problem – an overview

JANE SOMERVILLE

The subject of grown-up congenital heart disease is currently and correctly attracting attention in the world.

Surgical treatment for congenital heart disease (C.H.D) has evolved through the last 40 years, starting with the attempts by Blalock and Brock to palliate, to the current refined technical virtuoso repairs of the most complex in infancy. The explosive development of paediatric cardiology as a specialty has been inevitable, reaching maturity in 1980 with its own World Congress. In 1976 a unit for adolescent cardiac, medical and surgical cases was opened in the National Heart Hospital (N.H.H.), London, when the increasing and continuing demands of the young cardiac survivors with congenital malformations who had been treated in infancy and childhood were recognised.

Although the British Heart Foundation suggests in a 1989 advertisement that 90 percent of patients born with congenital heart disease survive to adulthood, calculations based on many assumptions suggest that the correct figure is closer to 60–70 percent. Looking at the numbers of adolescent cardiac admissions (aged 12–19 years) to the N.H.H. there was a steady increase until 1977 (Figure 1); thereafter there was a fall in absolute numbers which remain the same over the last decade. Ninety-five percent of these patients had congenital heart diseases and 75 percent had earlier palliative and/or reparative surgery. By the end of the 1980s the over-20s exceeded the adolescents and the over-30s are rising (Figure 2). Thus, the problem is *not* in provision for adolescents alone, it is for a whole large group, mainly adults. It is not a paediatric problem and most adolescents resent or refuse treatment as a child. The requirements for adolescent cardiac patients differ in the last decade compared to the 1970s (Table 1) and the reasons for admission to hospital of all grown-up C.H.D. are shown (Figure 3). The fall in adolescent cardiac requirements for In-Patient services relates to improved non-invasive technology (echocardiography and magnetic resonance imaging (M.R.I.) which diminish the need for invasive investigation, and probably with better surgery in the

1

John Hess and George R. Sutherland (eds.), Congenital Heart Disease in Adolescents and Adults, 1–13.
© 1992 *Kluwer Academic Publishers. Printed in the Netherlands.*

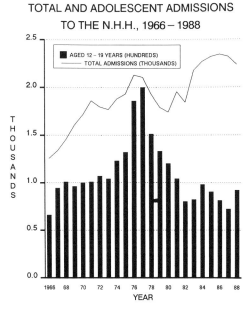

Figure 1. Total and adolescent (age 12–19 years) admissions to the National Heart Hospital, 1966–1988.

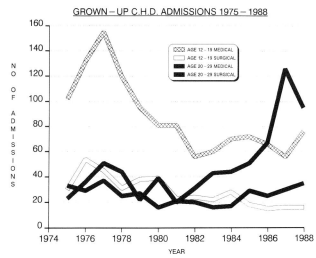

Figure 2. Graph to show the medical and surgical admissions to the National Heart Hospital of patients aged 12–19 years and 20–29 years with congenital heart disease from 1974–1988.

late 1970s and 1980s the serious problems may be reduced or delayed until later. Provision of day case facilities has diminished the requirements for In-Patient beds. Since patients come from long distances for such specialised facilities, day stays for full assessment and minor procedures are useful.

Table 1. The changing reasons for admission of adolescents/young adults with congenital heart disease. Facility for day cases started in 1984.

	Year of admission	
	1970–1979	1980–1989
Reason for admission		
Arrhythmias	19%	39%
Investigation	43%	18%
Intervention	–	8%
Endocarditis	9%	6%
Myocardial failure	18%	12%
Pulmonary hypertension	11%	5%
Transplant assessment	–	12%

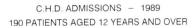

C.H.D. ADMISSIONS – 1989
190 PATIENTS AGED 12 YEARS AND OVER

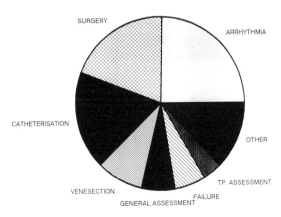

Figure 3. Pie to show reasons for admission of all adolescents and adults with congenital heart disease in 1989.

Medical (cardiology) demand for in-patient services

As can be seen from Table 1, arrhythmias, myocardial failure and transplant assessment, endocarditis, complication of pulmonary vascular disease and intervention with investigation make most of the claims on beds.

Arrhythmias

This is the commonest reason for admission in all decades, becoming more frequent with increasing age. Arrhythmias occur as part of the natural history of many anomalies, and after surgery the same and new arrhythmias may be delayed in their onset or induced prematurely. There may be a symptomatic deterioration from paroxysmal and/or established rhythm disorders requiring identification and correct therapy. The need to investigate and prevent sudden unexpected death is demanding on resources. Several points emerge from our experience of patients managed in and outside the special centre. Cardiologists, who rarely understand the underlying disorder, tend to ignore it and often use drugs which cause accelerated deterioration in the function of the already abnormal myocardium. Informed help tends to be sought only when disaster and irreversible problems have occurred. There is a temptation to control the rate of atrial flutter and fibrillation with drugs such as Amiodarone and Beta-Blockers and ignore the pressing need to restore sinus rhythm. There is a disquieting single-minded obsession to investigate and master ventricular arrhythmias as a cause of sudden death and ignore the role of atrial flutter. Atrial flutter is the commonest arrhythmia post Fontan, in single ventricle and tricuspid atresia and post-Mustard. It occurs often in Fallot, associated with right ventricular dysfunction and worsening it, and often is related to malfunctioning conduits. Three aborted 'sudden' deaths in this unit's series have been shown to have collapses due to subsequent atrial flutter, having been treated with the wrong drug due to the erroneous assumption that ventricular tachycardia was the cause. Sophistication is needed to differentiate atrial flutter with a one-to-one response in a patient with right bundle branch block, so frequently present in post surgical heart disease, from ventricular tachycardia. The adult cardiologist's knowledge and wisdom relating to management of arrhythmias must be united with the paediatric cardiologist's understanding of anatomy and post-operative complications. Too often the danger of the thromboembolic complication are ignored by paediatricians and thrombus often collects in the diseased fibrillating right atrium.

Serious problems may be encountered by patients needing pacemakers and recurrent changes. These should be performed by experts, not by junior staff in training. There may be a shortage of venous access and abnormality of drainage, special pacemaking needs such as a dual chamber which may induce flutter causing more symptoms, profound functional deterioration with pace-maker failures, and serious complications from sepsis have caused the death of a few long term survivors. Patients with heart block complicating their lesions have a worse long term outcome than their counterparts with sinus rhythm, even without pacemaker failure. This highlights the special importance and risks of pacing in grown-up congenital heart disease – it requires specialised experience.

Endocarditis

Despite instruction of patient and doctor, endocarditis occurs in post operative congenital heart disease (Table 2) as well as unoperated C.H.D. There are some lesions which are not 'attacked' by bacteria so prophylaxis is not instituted in these (Table 3). The major problem now faced is delayed diagnosis. Doctor and

Table 2. The basic lesions present in post-operative endocarditis after surgery for congenital heart disease – the majority were adolescents and adults.

Basic lesion	%
Left valves	65
T.G.A. (Rastelli)	4
V.S.D. (Open)	6
Fallot	8
Complex repairs	9
Cont. intra-operative infection	8

Table 3. Congenital cardiac lesions which do *not* require protection from infective endocarditis.

Pulmonary valve stenosis & post-op. valvotomy
Secundum/sinus venosus A.S.D.
Post-op. closed[a]:   A.S.D.
                       V.S.D.
                       Duct
Total anomalous pulmonary venous drainage
Removed cor triatriatum
Fallot, well repaired: No shunts, A.R., V.S.D.,
                         No valve grafts

[a]Provided no left valve abnormalities.
A.R. = aortic regurgitation; A.S.D. = atrial septal defect; V.S.D. = ventricular septal defect.

patient are aware of the risk, but doctors do not consider the possibility of the diagnosis and rarely initiate appropriate tests or referral, prior to giving antibiotics. The result of this attitude is D.D.D. (delay and destruction and disaster). Education is important and appears to fail to date. In recognising and highlighting the risk, one has a responsibility to point to the dangers of not making an early diagnosis and suppressing the disease by inadvisable therapy as well as the initiation of prophylaxis. The only hope is to educate the patients whose prime concern is for proper treatment of themselves.

Terminal and transplant assessment

Myocardial failure may result from a residual lesion, damage to the myocardium sustained during early/long bypasses, or from congenital abnormality of the myocardium as part of diffuse congenital cardiovascular disease over and above the compensatory hypertrophy and dilatation. Prior to 1975, myocardial protection during bypass was inadequate, damage occurred from potassium arrests, bad technique and long operations without adequate or any coronary perfusion. When patients survived, healing fibrosis and even excessive endocardial fibrosis looking like fibroelastosis can occur as late sequelae, probably the result of sub-endocardial ischaemia during bypass. This is very uncommon now. However, terminal failure patients collect in a specialised unit hoping for heart or heart/lung transplant. Such patients use many resources and as a result of shortages in finance and personnel may prevent less hopeless routine problems being solved. Patients are accepted for transplant (which they may never get) and the emotional and medical support must be provided by the unit. Probably 85 percent of early Mustards, many Fontan patients, most univentricular hearts and many other malformations will need this before 30 years if survival is to be prolonged.

Surgical demands

Cardiac surgery is still and increasingly required for congenital heart disease in adolescents and adults. The type of surgery required has changed over the last decade (Figure 4) with increasing needs for re-operation on the definitive repair and decreasing requirement for first radical repairs, as expected. The needs continue to the fourth decade and presumably will continue for longer (Figure 5). Re-operations are mainly for degeneration in valves and conduits and native valves; this involves most patients who have had 'repair' using conduits and valves and covers many complex malformations. Endocarditis and new lesions may require reoperation. The morbidity and mortality may be high. Parents and patients should be warned of the need in the future and not be dispatched during childhood with the belief that they are 'cured' for all time. Many problems are encountered and 're-opening', which may be associated with catastrophe, must be performed by the experienced. Undoubtedly this will change, but the need for surgical expertise will remain. The cardiac surgical expertise in the older congenitals will be required to help with the coronary artery disease which will be acquired by many late survivors – a problem that is now appearing in 40 and 50 year olds, operated on in childhood.

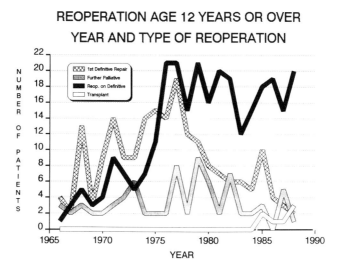

Figure 4. Graph to show type of reoperation required for congenital heart disease in adolescents and adults aged over 12 years.

REOPERATION FOR C.H.D.

PATIENTS AGED 12 YEARS AND OVER

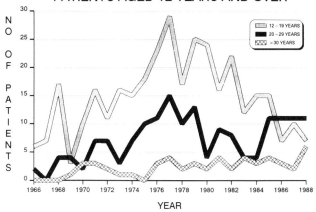

Figure 5. Age of patients with congenital heart disease needing reoperation 1966–1988.

Cardiologists looking after post-operative patients have a responsibility to refer patients back for surgery before serious deterioration in myocardial function – so often they do not do this. Right sided obstruction does not usually produce symptoms until serious and sometimes irreversible failure has occurred. Recognition of important obstruction may not be easy in this setting and requires understanding of subtleties, like the management of arrhythmias. Unfortunately, cardiologists often do not seek expert help. They must accept the responsibility of reading the operation report, know the natural history of the valves or conduit, know how to identify obstruction and refer at the correct time. Referral too late means a high operative mortality. The mortality for 'redo' Fontan is 44 percent, currently (Table 4). Undoubtedly this is

Table 4. Re-operation age 12 years and over for congenital heart disease. First re-operation on definitive repair.

Lesion	No.	Op. death
AVS	59	6(10%)
Fallot	26	3(12%)
RVOT reconstr.	26	2(8%)
Fontan	18	8(44%)
VSD/AR	17	4(24%)
Subaortic st.	13	2(15%)
Coarctation	13	0

AVS = aortic valve stenosis; No. = number; Op. = operative; Reconstr. = reconstruction; St. = stenosis; VSD/AR = ventricular septal defect and aortic regurgitation.

contributed to by errors of selection and technique, as well as late referral; some of the mortality can be avoided but this figure suggests that there is a problem which other units should recognise when they are undertaking both the first and subsequent operations. The urgent need for research into preventing or delaying calcification of biological valves cannot be over stressed.

It must be accepted that as techniques have improved, the residual and late problems change. Today's problems will not be tomorrow's, but cardiac surgical expertise is and will be needed for the grown-up congenital heart disease. How, where and by whom with what training requires to be addressed by the cardiac surgical hierarchy.

Out-patient support services

As can be predicted there are increasing Out-Patient referrals and problems as each decade's survivors are added to the next. Besides the cardiological problems, patients both well and ill seek advice about normal life's activities and demands in relation to their heart condition (Table 5). It is important that advice is given by the informed since bad management may contribute to loss of life or function. The general surgeon often fails to seek advice and the physician is called too late after an unnecessary serious complication. The plastic surgeon may be needed to even the incised breast or reduce deforming scars. Health insurance for these patients is going to be a problem for the future and very important with the decline of National Health Services. Life Insurance companies in the U.K. appear disinterested unless the sums are large and then the patient is refused or excessively loaded. Support clinics for 'at-risk' pregnancy, transoesophageal echocardiography, foetal scanning and pre/post transplant are needed once a service for grown-up congenital heart disease is established. Support for the bereaved family is demanded from the physician who takes over the care; families may return for up to 3 years after the death.

Table 5. Problems faced by patients with congenital heart disease.

Insurance
Pregnancy
Risk of affected offspring
Driving licences (ordinary or vocational)
Employment
Housing priority
Social service support
Contraception
Prison management and sentences
Psychological problems in relation to their heart disease

Who knows? Who cares?

The organisation for long term care of these patients is required now in any country which has had established effective cardiac surgery for infants and children over the last 20 years. Unfortunately the answer to Who Knows? is uncertain. Many patients come back to the surgeon whose name they remember, unlike that of the paediatric cardiologist! However surgeon's knowledge of late problems are concerned with mortality and reoperation with a common assumption that the rest are 'well'. The paediatric cardiologist is familiar with patients and underlying anomaly but unfamiliar with the one-to-one relationship with adult patients, the different cardiac problems encountered as an adult, drug regimes, and the management of the coronary heart disease and hypertension which will be acquired by some. An additional difficulty is that most paediatric cardiologists do not have access and/or control of adult In-Patient beds. The local cardiologist, to whom these patients are often referred by general practitioners and physicians, is usually ignorant of the underlying condition and its complications, see only the management of rhythm disorders and failure in routine cardiological terms, and tend to refer back for operations too late and with a reluctance (arrogance?) to seek help from the few informed sources. The patients will hopefully spend most of their lives as adults. To improve their care, the subject should be one of the subspecialities of cardiology, like electrophysiology, intervention or echocardiography. Special education of a few cardiologists and enthusiasm are vital, as well as the recognition that in most countries these patients are getting inadequate care. Some paediatric cardiologists already have enough experience in adult cardiology in their training and practice (recommended in the U.K. as a minimum of six months for the training of a paediatric cardiologist): they must organise adequate In-Patient facilities and integrate with the department of cardiology.

In managing grown-up C.H.D., a knowledge of prognosis and well-being of patients after the first decade of follow-up is needed. For this an ability index has been created [1] (Table 6). The index has taken into account the patient's perception of normality of life, as well as the doctor's! It is not only concerned with exercise tolerance and thus has more relevance than the N.Y.H.A. classification, as well as more colour! For ease of lecturing it has been colour coded by the readily remembered colours of the rainbow and is thus useful for quick comparison of results, saving verbose description.

It is also important to know the incidence and which special troublesome complications (Figures 6A & 6B) occur in the various conditions. This is useful for counselling, prevention of problems, and advice on way of life for the young. The incidence of late serious problems differs according to diseases and procedures and the surgeon (Figure 7) – a factor which is rarely considered. One Unit's results are not the same as anothers and nor are the late complications. With experience one can often tell where a Fallot's tetralogy has had repair by the residual lesions and problems!

Table 6. A new classification to define the capability of patients to lead a normal or restricted life, taking into account their adaptation to having or having had congenital heart disease. Description of Ability index (1–4) colour coded for easy demonstration.

Red	①	Normal live. Full time work or school. Manage pregnancy.
Yellow	②	Able to work. Intermittent symptoms. Interference with life.[a] Pregnancy possible.
Green	③	Unable to work. Limitation all activities. Pregnancy Risk.
Purple	④	Extreme limitation. Dependent. Almost housebound.

[a]Socio/community imposition because cardiac anomaly.

Organisation

Integrated with the proper provision of medical expertise is the basic oganisation and support services for long term care of the grown-up congenital heart disease patient. The *ROCK* concept has been designed for this:

– *R*ecognise the problem – paediatric cardiologist, parent and patient take responsibility.
– *O*rganise referral where there is or will be expertise. This must be flexible according to where the patient has come from i.e.: special cardiac centre, children's hospital or university clinic. Paediatric cardiologists must be the major people responsible for this organisation and referral. They may chose and/or train interested cardiological colleagues or do joint clinics. It must be decided and known where all original notes will be for that patients life. The current policy of note destruction in many centres of the U.K. (including our own), particularly if patients are not seen for 10 years, is jeopardising optimal care.
– *C*entralise the specialist needs and expensive technology in a few centres, i.e. 4–5 for U.K. Facilities should not be diluted by every cardiac centre wanting to 'have a go', There are relatively few patients and expertise, particularly in the tough problems, will be hard to acquire if there is dissipation and small mumbers.
– *K*nowledge which is centralised must include the listed skills (Table 7).

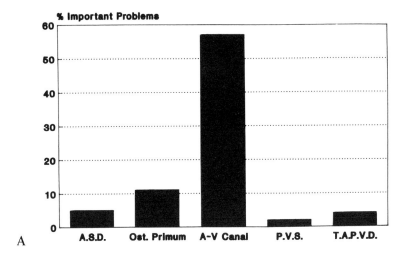

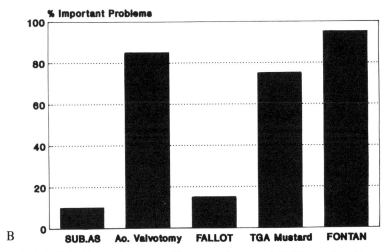

Figure 6. A & B: Incidence of major problems in patients aged 12–20 years in different types of congenital heart disease operated on after a decade of follow-up. Major problems referred to are death, reoperation, endocarditis, symptomatic arrhythmia, or Ability Index 3/4.

Currently in Europe there are few centres, less than 10, who have organised proper care and supervision, and even fewer trained cardiologists with the appropriate knowledge. A survey done through the members of the A.E.P.C. confirms this state of chaos. However, judging from the plenary sessions and state of the art lectures sought, European cardiology as well as Japan, U.S.A. and Turkey are gradually stirring and their awareness must be the start.

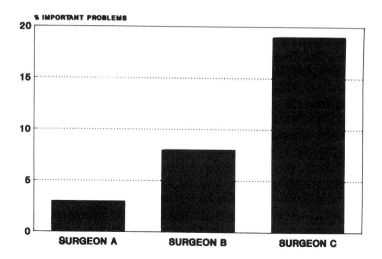

Figure 7. Incidence of important late problems according to which surgeon performed the operation of radical repair of Fallot's tetralogy, operated on age 2–10 years.

Table 7. Knowledge/Skills required to be centralized for optimal management of 'grown-up' congenital heart disease.

Adult congenital heart disease ⎫
Acquired heart disease   ⎬ Cardiologist
Echo/magnetic resonance imaging
Invasive investigation/intervention
Expert cardiac surgery
Arrhythmia management
[Transplant]

Conclusion

As can be seen there is much mork to be done for the 'grown-up' congenital heart patients. This new medical community has evolved from the dramatic progress of medicine and surgery. The welfare and needs of the patient (not status and wishes of individuals, physicians or organisations) must be the first consideration. Already medical society has lavished expert care, technology, and finance to ensure their survival. This responsibility cannot be relinquished once they reach adult life, they deserve our professional best and long term concern.

Acknowledgements

Without Sue Stone, my Research Assistant who controls the computer and the author, this work could not have been done. I thank Dr. and Mrs. Milton Paul for recording the lecture so that I could remember what I said!

References

1. Warnes C, Somerville J. Tricuspid atresia in adolescents and adults: Current state and late complications. Br. Heart J. 1986; 56:535–43.

2. Pulmonary vascular disease in congenital heart disease in adults

C.A. WAGENVOORT

Introduction

There is a considerable variety of pulmonary vascular diseases but none of these is pathognomonic for any particular congenital heart disease. Lung vessels react to chemical, physical or haemodynamic agents and stimuli in various ways. Usually this happens with a combination of lesions which form a characteristic pattern. Often these patterns are associated with pulmonary hypertension but not necessarily so. These patterns are far from aetiologic entities, although in each of them there is most likely a single pathogenesis. Therefore, various congenital cardiac defects that have little in common, may be accompanied by the same type of pulmonary vascular disease, as long as they produce the same haemodynamic disturbances. Also acquired cardiac or non-cardiac conditions with similar haemodynamics are associated with the same pattern of lesions in the lung vessels. From a lung biopsy specimen, the pathologist, though unable to diagnose any specific cardiac disease or malformation, can identify a distinct group of conditions which may be very helpful for establishing the clinical diagnosis.

Pulmonary vascular disease due to congenital heart disease, is not essentially different in adults and children. However, there are marked gradual differences related to their severity, chance of progression or reversibility and chance of complicating vascular alterations. Obviously, this has consequences for the prognosis and for the outlook as regards corrective surgery or other treatment. There is hardly any form of pulmonary vascular disease that occurs exclusively in children or exclusively in adults. Here the discussions will be limited to those types of pulmonary vascular disease that are likely to occur in adult patients with congenital heart disease. This applies to the patterns of lesions characteristically associated with the various cardiac anomalies or to complicating vascular alterations (Table 1).

John Hess and George R. Sutherland (eds.), Congenital Heart Disease in Adolescents and Adults, 15–33.
© *1992 Kluwer Academic Publishers. Printed in the Netherlands.*

Table 1.

Plexogenic arteriopathy:	pre-tricuspid shunt – A.S.D.
	post-tricuspid shunt – V.S.D.,
	P.D.A.
Congestive vasculopathy:	congenital aortic stenosis
	congenital mitral insufficiency
	(sometimes complicating
	other patterns when there is
	left ventricular failure)
Vasculopathy in diminished flow and pulse pressure:	tetralogy of Fallot
Thrombotic arteriopathy:	may complicate other patterns
	(occurs also as independent
	vascular disease)

Patterns of pulmonary vascular lesions associated with or complicating various types of congenital heart disease in adults. (A.S.D. = arterial septal defect; V.S.D. = ventricular septal defect; P.D.A. = patent ductus arteriosus).

Plexogenic arteriopathy

Aetiology and pathogenesis

Plexogenic arteriopathy is a morphologic and almost certainly also a pathogenetic entity. There is much evidence that intense vasoconstriction is the main, although probably not the only, pathogenetic factor. The aetiology of this spastic vasoconstriction, however, is very diverse. Plexogenic arteriopathy has developed in response to antiappetizer drugs and, although rarely, in association with hepatic disease; the latter cause may also be responsible for its occurrence in visceral schistosomiasis. It also occurs as a primary form without any detectable cause. It is likely that in these patients a hyperreactivity of the pulmonary arterial bed is involved. The most common cause is congenital heart disease with a left-to-right shunt, either a pretricuspid shunt as in atrial septal defect, or a posttricuspid shunt as in ventricular septal defect or patent ductus arteriosus. It is likely that not only in primary, but also in the various secondary forms of plexogenic arteriopathy, an individual degree of pulmonary arterial reactivity will determine the severity and progression of the vascular disease.

Morphology

There is a sequence of vascular changes in plexogenic arteriopathy (Table 2) [1,2]. When this condition is associated with a congenital cardiac shunt, this sequence starts at birth and the first alteration is an increased muscularity of

Table 2.

1. medial hypertrophy and muscularization of arterioles
2. cellular proliferation of the intima
3. concentric – laminar intimal fibrosis
4. dilatation lesions
5. fibrinoid necrosis
6. plexiform lesions

Arterial lesions of plexogenic arteriopathy in sequential order: 1 and 2 are reversible, 5 and 6 irreversible; of 3 and 4, the mild forms are in principle reversible, the severe forms irreversible.

the pulmonary arterial tree. This increase can be recognized in two forms. The media or muscular coat of the muscular pulmonary arteries becomes thicker and peripheral branches, normally devoid of muscle, develop a complete media with smooth muscle cells wedged between two elastic laminae.

Medial hypertrophy and *muscularization of arterioles* (Figure 1) are virtually always present whenever there is a shunt of any significance. In infants and in most young children these are the only vascular alterations.

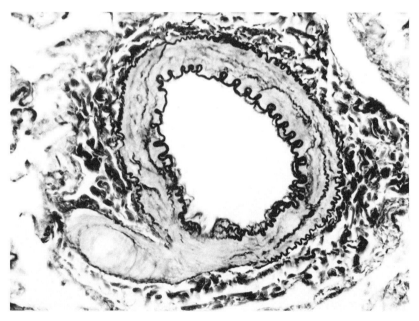

Figure 1. Muscular pulmonary artery in plexogenic arteriopathy. There is pronounced medial hypertrophy, while an arteriole is muscularized (ElvG, × 230).

In a pretricuspid shunt, increased muscularity of pulmonary arteries often remains the only change. In adult patients, however, complicating intimal lesions may occur or even the complete scala of plexogenic arteriopathy in the rare event of hyperreactive lung vessels.

In posttricuspid shunts, intimal thickening may occur. It begins with *cellular proliferation of the intima* which in arteries of small calibre may cause considerable narrowing of the lumen (Figure 2). The proliferating cells are derived from the media and ther muscular origin is usually still recognizable in electronmicroscopic preparations. Gradually collagen fibres are deposited between the cells and in later stages also elastic fibres, the latter sometimes in abundance. The intimal fibrosis developed in this way is peculiar in that it consists of concentric layers with an onion skin configuration (Figure 3). This *concentric-laminar intimal fibrosis* is clearly recognizable not only in an elastic stain but also in a haematoxylin stain. It may lead to complete obliteration of the lumen and, certainly when it is prominent, indicates severe pulmonary hypertension.

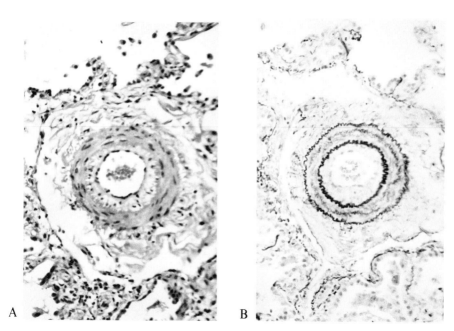

A   B

Figure 2. Muscular pulmonary artery in plexogenic arteriopathy with medial hypertrophy and cellular intimal proliferation (A: H&E; B: ElvG; both × 240).

In the last stages of the disease, *dilatation lesions* occur in the form of wide, thin-walled, so-called vein-like branches of muscular arteries (Figure 4), or in clusters of such branches [3].

Occasionally these clusters become very large to form angiomatoid lesions. Moreover, the proximal part of a branch, shortly after its origin from a larger artery, may become the site of *fibrinoid necrosis* of the vascular wall (Figure 5). It is usually associated with a clot of fibrin and platelets in the lumen. Focal dilation in this area together with recanalization of this clot produces the very characteristic *plexiform lesion*. The plexus in the centre consists of

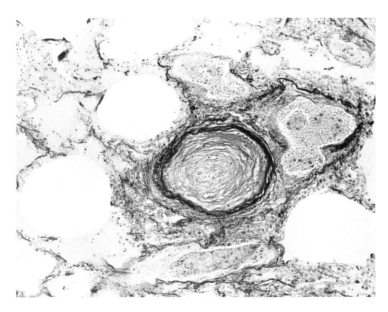

Figure 3. Pulmonary artery in plexogenic arteriopathy with complete obliteration by concentric-laminar intimal fibrosis (ElvG, × 60).

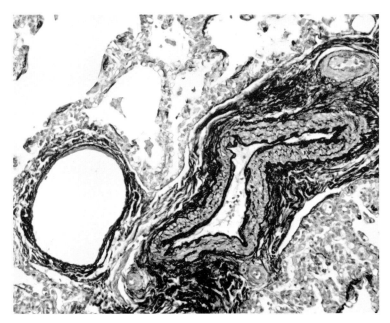

Figure 4. Pulmonary artery in plexogenic arteriopathy with two branches. One (top right) is muscularized, the other (bottom left) shows a dilatation lesion with loss of virtually all smooth muscle (ElvG, × 150).

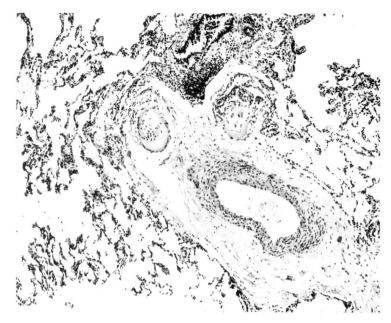

Figure 5. Pulmonary artery in plexogenic arteriopathy with two branches, both with fibrinoid necrosis. The branch at right also contains an incipient plexiform lesion (H&E, × 60).

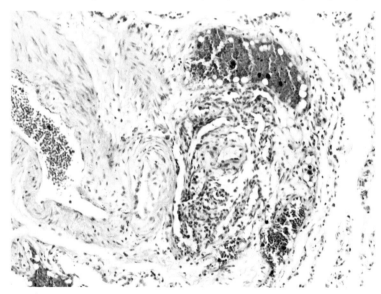

Figure 6. Pulmonary artery with plexiform lesion; on top of this there is a thin-walled dilated branch (H&E, × 150).

capillary-like channels, separated by cells with hyperchromatic nuclei. Distal to the plexus there are one or more dilated thin-walled branches (Figure 6).

Reversibility and prognosis

From lung biopsies taken during open heart surgery and by checking the follow-up of a patient with for instance a ventricular septal defect, considerable experience has been gained with regard to the reversibility or irreversibility of the various lesions. In a number of patients, with severe pulmonary hypertension, in whom a banding of the pulmonary artery was performed, it was even possible to compare the vascular morphology in two biopsies taken at the time of the banding and some years later during corrective surgery respectively [4].

In this way it could be demonstrated that, when the cause of the pulmonary hypertension is removed by closing the shunt, medial hypertrophy is reversible. The increased muscularity regresses often to normal but anyhow to a significant degree. The same is true for cellular intimal proliferation even when this appeared very extensive in the first lung biopsy; a thin collagen-rich fibrotic layer may be the only remnant. It is different when concentric-laminar intimal fibrosis has developed. This will regress when it is mild but not when it is severe. As far as could be ascertained a similar situation exists with dilatation lesions. The vein-like branches often seem to regress but the clusters of thin-walled vessels, certainly when they are large, show no such tendency. Fibrinoid necrosis and plexiform lesions, when found in a biopsy specimen, carry a very ominous prognosis. It is even so that, whenever there are severe changes such as prominent concentric-laminar intimal fibrosis and dilatation lesions or fibrinoid necrosis and plexiform lesions, there is not only no regression but progression of the vascular disease. These patients are greatly at risk during or immediately following corrective surgery but even when they survive this period, they may develop intractable pulmonary hypertension, months or years later.

Special relevance to adult patients

Plexogenic arteriopathy is particularly observed in children, since surgical correction of congenital cardiac disease is mostly carried out at an early age. There are, however, exceptions. One group concerns patients with an atrial septal defect, who are first examined and treated in adult life, since in this condition symptoms often start late. Usually only the mild stages of plexogenic arteriopathy, not beyond an increased muscularity, are observed in atrial septal defect. Often medial hypertrophy is not recognized because the lung vessels are dilated to accomodate the prominently increased pulmonary flow that prevails in this condition. Pulmonary arterial dilation causes the thick media to become thinner so that the ratio between medial thickness and external vascular diameter becomes normal. A true increase in pulmonary arterial smooth muscle can be demonstrated in these cases by assessing the total surface area of arterial media's in relation to the surface area of lung tissue in which these vessels are found [5].

This arterial dilation is generalized and uniform. It also affects capillaries and veins. It is unrelated to dilatation lesions. In fact, it is not a lesion but an adaptation to the large flow. Morphometry, outlined above, is a very laborious and time consuming way of establishing arterial dilation in these instances. There is an easier, though less reliable method to detect arterial dilation in atrial septal defect. This means comparing the calibre of the pulmonary artery with the bronchus it accompanies. Normally the artery is somewhat smaller than, or at most similar in size to the bronchus it is associated with, but during dilation it will become much larger (Figure 7). Bronchi, however, may constrict or collapse so that the method has to be applied with great care. Only very significant dilation of arteries can be identified in this way.

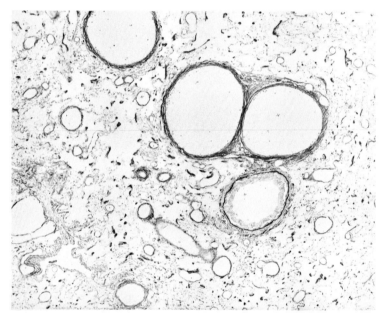

Figure 7. Generalized dilation of pulmonary arteries in atrial septal defect. Also pulmonary veins, near left lower corner, are wide (ElvG, × 60).

Intimal fibrosis may occur in adult patients with atrial septal defect. It is usually limited to mild intimal thickening which is not of the concentric-laminar type but which must be regarded as an age change or as incidental postthrombotic lesions. These changes have no or little clinical significance. However, in a small group of adult patients with atrial septal defect, advanced and progressive plexogenic arteriopathy develops with all its consequences. It is not clear why this happens in these unfortunate few, but it seems likely that this is a group of patients with hyperreactive lung vessels, so that this secondary form of pulmonary hypertension is closely akin to primary plexogenic arteriopathy.

Patients with post-tricuspid shunts are far more likely to die in childhood or adolescence, either during operation or, if unoperated, from severe pulmonary hypertension. In patients who reach adulthood with an Eisenmenger syndrome, the most advanced lesions of plexogenic arteriopathy are likely to be present in their pulmonary vasculature, although there is the occasional exception. In most young patients with congenital heart disease, who have fibrinoid necrosis and/or plexiform lesions, a fatal outcome within one to three years is likely. In those who reach adult life with such arterial alterations, progression often slows down so that they may live on till well in their fourth decade or beyond.

Postthrombotic changes in the form of eccentric intimal fibrosis, intimal plaques with recanalization channels or intravascular septa may complicate plexogenic arteriopathy particularly in adult patients.

Signs of congestive vasculopathy, particularly alterations in the pulmonary veins may sometimes occur when there is for instance mitral regurgitation as often in atrioventricular septal defect or in the presence of left ventricular failure.

Congestive vasculopathy

Aetiology and pathogenesis

One of the most common forms of hypertensive pulmonary vascular disease is due to chronic congestion of the lung. While an elevation of the pressure in the pulmonary veins is the single most important pathogenetic factor, the aetiology is greatly varied. Some of the many conditions that cause an impediment to pulmonary venous outflow and that thus may give rise to pulmonary venous hypertension, are very common.

The obstruction to the venous flow may be localized in large pulmonary venous trunks, either by congenital stenosis or resulting from outside pressure by tumour or other processes. Idiopathic mediastinal fibrosis is a well-known example. Obstruction at left atrial level may be observed in cor triatriatum or in the presence or a left atrial myxoma and a similar effect may be produced by mitral stenosis and incompetence, whether congenital or acquired. Most frequently congestive vasculopathy is seen when the problem is in the left ventricle. Aortic stenosis and incompetence, systemic hypertension, coronary heart disease and myocardial disease, may all produce this pattern of lesions. Intermittent bouts of pulmonary venous pressure elevation have an effect similar to that of continuous elevation. This may explain that congestive vasculopathy is often seen in patients who never experienced clear left ventricular failure.

Morpholopy

In congestive vasculopathy all lung vessels may be affected: pulmonary arteries, capillaries and veins. Usually some changes can be found in the lymphatics and, in a number of cases, the lung tissue is also involved (Table 3) [1].

Table 3.

A. Pulmonary arteries:	(often severe) medial thickening[a] muscularization of arterioles eccentric, non-laminar, non-obliterating intimal fibrosis[a]
B. Pulmonary veins:	medial thickening[a] arterialization (mild) intimal fibrosis[a]
C. Lung tissue:	haemosiderosis (often) interstitial fibrosis[a]
D. Lymphatics:	dilation

Vascular and parenchymal changes in congestive vasculopathy. The vascular lesions are potentially reversible.
[a]Partly due to interstitial oedema and fibrosis.

The *muscular pulmonary arteries* tend to show thickening of the media, which may be very pronounced and is usually accompanied by muscularization of arterioles (Figure 8). Particularly in adults, the medial thickening appears to result in part from interstitial oedema and fibrosis, so that it is not a reliable yardstick for arterial muscularity [6]. This may explain that there is often a poor correlation between the degree of medial hypertrophy and the pulmonary arterial pressure and resistance.

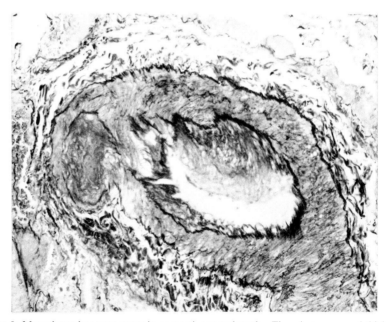

Figure 8. Muscular pulmonary artery in congestive vasculopathy. There is pronounced thickening of the media and intimal fibrosis both accentuated by interstitial oedema (ElvG, × 230).

Interstitial oedema also plays a part in thickening of adventitia and intima. Intimal fibrosis may be pronounced in congestive vasculopathy so that the lumen of muscular pulmonary arteries is greatly narrowed over long stretches (Figure 9). It is usually eccentric but even if circumferential, it does not have an onionskin appearance. Complete obliteration, does not occur and recanalization of the intimal patches is rare. Arteritis is uncommon; fibrinoid necrosis, dilatation lesions and plexiform lesions are absent.

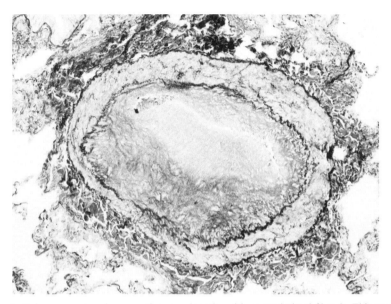

Figure 9. Pulmonary artery in congestive vasculopathy with severe intimal fibrosis. This provides narrowing but not obliteration of the lumen (ElvG, × 230).

Thickening of the media of *pulmonary veins* is common and sometimes very striking. Moreover, the haphazard arrangement of elastic fibres in their walls changes to distinct internal and external elastic laminae. As a consequence the venous wall resembles that of an artery: arterialization of pulmonary veins (Figure 10). Intimal fibrosis of pulmonary veins is common but usually mild.

At an ultrastructural level it appears that the walls of *pulmonary capillaries* are thickened; this may be accompanied by interstitial fibrosis of the *lung tissue*. Iron pigment is usually deposited in lung tissue as focal or diffuse haemosiderosis. The *lymphatics* of the lung are generally dilated.

Reversibility and prognosis

Our information about reversibility of congestive vasculopathy is based almost exclusively upon acquired cardiac disease, particularly upon rheumatic mitral stenosis. Generally speaking, it seems justified to apply the same data to patients with congenital heart disease.

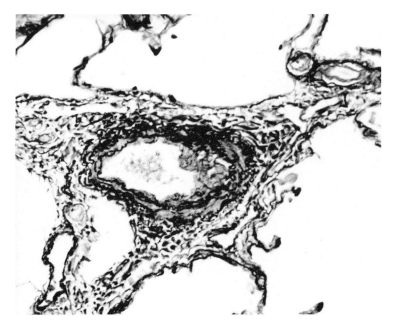

Figure 10. Pulmonary vein in congestive vasculopathy with thickening of media and reduplication of elastic lamina (arterialization) (ElvG, × 230).

Upon relief of a mitral stenosis, there may be such a sudden decrease in pulmonary arterial pressure that it is disproportional to the pronounced vascular changes with severe narrowing of lumens in a lung biopsy specimen, taken during valvotomy or valve replacement. This almost certainly is due to marked interstitial oedema which may disappear rapidly upon removal of the impediment to the pulmonary venous outflow. Long term regression has also been demonstrated, even to the extent that prominent medial thickness and intimal fibrosis may disappear almost completely [1,7].

Special relevance to adult patients

It has been assumed that there are no differences in congestive pulmonary vascular pathology between patients with acquired and those with congenital heart disease. While this is likely to be true, it does not apply to age. There are, at least in acquired congestive vasculopathy significant differences between adults and children with rheumatic mitral stenosis as studies in India have shown. In children, pulmonary hypertension is often progressively severe with a poorer prognosis than in adults [8]. In the muscular pulmonary arteries of these children there is hardly any intimal fibrosis but a very thick media, without interstitial oedema or fibrosis, indicating a markedly increased muscularity [6]. Particularly in children and adolescents there is a reasonable correlation between pulmonary vascular changes and pulmonary arterial pressure and resistance [9]. Such a correlation is absent or very poor in adults. For that reason, in adults a pre-operative biopsy in order to decide whether the pulmonary vasculature will allow corrective heart surgery, is rarely if at all necessary.

Vasculopathy in diminished flow and pulse pressure

Aetiology and pathogenesis

This pattern of pulmonary vascular lesions occurs in patients with tetralogy of Fallot or related forms of cyanotic congenital heart disease. The decreased pulse pressure due to the pulmonic stenosis, has a prominent effect on the muscularity of the pulmonary arteries. In these cyanotic patients the haematocrit is increased as is the total blood volume. One of the effects is an increased tendency to thrombosis, particularly of pulmonary arteries (Table 4).

Table 4.

1. Medial atrophy
2. Widening of all lung vessels
3. Thrombotic lesions; delicate septa
4. Collateral vessels and anastomoses

Vascular lesions in cases of diminished flow and pulse pressure.

Morphology

In patients with tetralogy of Fallot the muscular pulmonary arteries are wide and thin-walled (Figure 11). The muscular coat not only becomes atrophic but even in medium-sized arteries all smooth muscle may disappear. It is likely that an increased blood volume in combination with the flabby vascular walls, is responsible for the increased width of the lumen.

Not only the arteries, but also the alveolar capillaries and the pulmonary veins are dilated. The veins are even more thin-walled than normal.

Thrombotic changes are common in tetralogy of Fallot. In a number of patients they are abundant. Recent and old thrombi with various stages of organization and recanalization, may be found in numerous muscular pulmonary arteries (Figure 12). Intravascular septa, resulting from recanalization, are especially striking because the generalized increase of luminal width applies also to the recanalization channels. This is turn results in very delicate septa (Figure 13). It is remarkable that these thrombotic changes are scarce or absent in pulmonary veins.

There is usually an extensive collateral circulation in tetralogy of Fallot, witnessed by enlarged bronchial arteries and by the development of multiple systemic arterial branches in pleura and interlobular septa. As all systemic

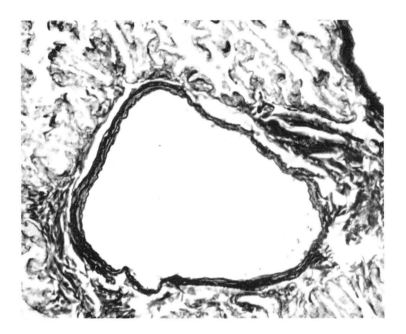

Figure 11. Wide and thin-walled pulmonary artery in tetralogy of Fallot. In parts of the circumference all smooth muscle has disappeared (ElvG, ×230).

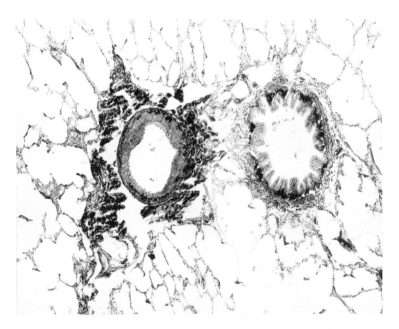

Figure 12. Pulmonary artery in tetralogy of Fallot, with irregular, eccentric intimal fibrosis and thin media (ElvG, ×60).

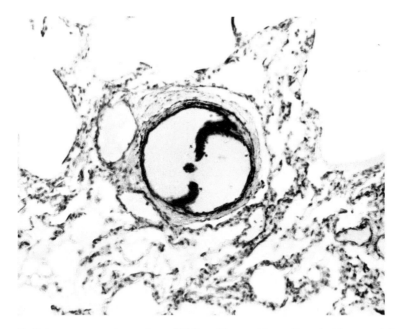

Figure 13. Pulmonary artery in tetralogy of Fallot with very thin media and with tangentially cut intravascular septa (ElvG, × 230).

arteries, they have a distinct internal elastic lamina but no external lamina, as in pulmonary arteries. Anastomoses between systemic and pulmonary arteries, though difficult to visualize, are common.

Reversibility and prognosis

Not much is known about reversibility of the various pulmonary vascular changes in tetralogy of Fallot. In rare instances in which a lung biopsy specimen was taken during surgical correction of the cardiac defect and could be compared with autopsy material when the patient died at a later stage, width and wall thickness of the arteries seemed to have returned to normal. It has been claimed, that postthrombotic lesions, including the intravascular septa, disappear following the creation of a Blalock anastomosis or other surgical shunt [10]. This certainly happens not always. If such a shunt is too large, plexogenic arteriopathy may develop with all its consequences. The combination of plexiform lesions with intravascular septa, apparently dating from a pre-operative period, has been reported.

Special relevance to adult patients

Although thinning of the media of pulmonary arteries and even thrombotic changes have been reported in infants [11], there is no doubt that all alterations are far more prominent in adolescents and adults. This is particularly true for post-thrombotic changes such as the intravascular septa. These septa may be so abundant in adult patients that one would expect that following correction of the cardiac defect, pulmonary hypertension would develop, as a result of the generalized vascular obstruction. However, it appears that this is a very rare event.

Thrombotic arteriopathy

Definition and incidence

Vascular lesions that are the sequelae of thrombi, are extraordinarily common. They occur in small numbers in the great majority of normal, healthy individuals over the age of 50 years and often in much younger persons. Of course, in these instances we should speak of 'post-thrombotic lesions' and not of 'thrombotic arteriopathy', since these isolated changes have no clinical significance. There are, however, many conditions, particularly lung and heart diseases, including congenital cardiac anomalies, that may become complicated by postthrombotic lesions on a far greater scale. In a number of these cases it is appropriate to speak of 'complicating thrombotic arteriopathy' since it is likely that these pulmonary vascular alterations may produce symptoms or may aggravate the symptoms of the original disease.

Thrombotic arteriopathy also occurs as an independent disease, that ultimately may lead to severe pulmonary hypertension, right ventricular failure and death. This may be the result of repeated bouts of thromboembolism but there is little doubt that is can also occur on the basis of primary thrombosis of small pulmonary arteries. A problem for the pathologist is that thromboemboli and primary thrombi cannot be distinguished histologically.

Morphology and reversibility

Recent thrombi are almost always uncommon, even in conditions associated with severe pulmonary hypertension. Organization of thrombi leads to eccentric patches of intimal fibrosis (Figure 14) and relatively often to complete obliteration of the lumen, usually over short stretches. Recanalization is common (Figure 15). It occurs in the form of capillaries or one or two large channels equipped with a muscular coat. Multiple wide channels are associated with intravascular septa (Figure 16). The changes are essentially the same as those observed in tetralogy of Fallot but the septa are usually far more coarse.

Special relevance to adult patients

In young patients with congenital heart disease such as ventricular septal defect, the various lesions of thrombotic arteriopathy are more common than in normal individuals. The incidence of these lesions increases, however, with

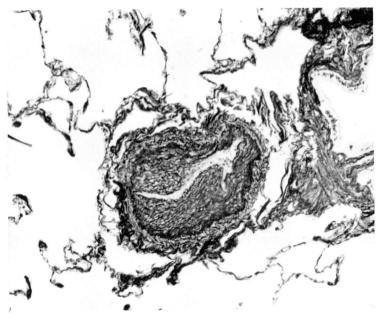

Figure 14. Pulmonary artery with severe eccentric, postthrombotic intimal fibrosis, complicating a case of plexogenic arteriopathy (ElvG, ×150).

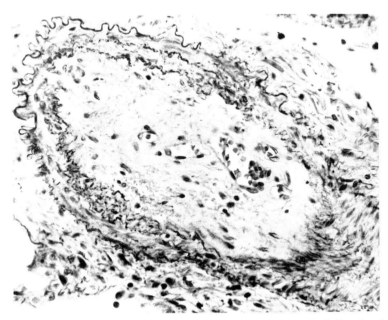

Figure 15. Pulmonary artery with obliteration by postthrombotic intimal fibrosis, showing recanalization by capillary-like channels (ElvG, ×230).

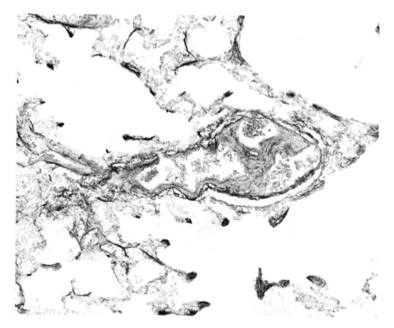

Figure 16. Pulmonary artery in thrombotic arteriopathy. Recanalization of postthrombotic intimal fibrosis resulted in wide channels and intravascular septa (ElvG, × 150).

age. In adults with congenital heart disease of any type, the number of postthrombotic lesions rises sharply particularly after the age of 40 years. There is little doubt that in some cases these changes contribute to an existing pulmonary hypertension. The rôle of thrombosis in adult patients with tetralogy of Fallot, has been discussed above.

References

1. Wagenvoort CA, Mooi WJ. Biopsy pathology of the pulmonary vasculature. London: Chapman & Hall, 1989.
2. Edwards WD. The pathology of secondary pulmonary hypertension. In: Fishman AP, editor. The pulmonary circulation: Normal and abnormal. Philadelphia: Univ Pennsylv Press, 1990: 329–42.
3. Heath D, Edwards JE. The pathology of hypertensive pulmonary vascular disease: A description of six grades of structural changes in the pulmonary arteries with special reference to congenital cardiac defects. Circulation 1958; 18:533–47.
4. Wagenvoort CA, Wagenvoort N, Draulans-Noë Y. Reversibility of plexogenic pulmonary arteriopathy following banding of the pulmonary artery. J Thorac Cardiovasc Surg 1984; 87:876–86.
5. Wagenvoort CA. Vasoconstriction and medial hypertrophy in pulmonary hypertension. Circulation 1960; 22:535–46.
6. Wagenvoort CA, Wagenvoort N. Smooth muscle content of pulmonary arterial media in pulmonary venous hypertension compared with other forms of pulmonary hypertension. Chest 1982; 81:581–5.

7. Ramirez A, Grimes ET, Abelmann WH. Regression of pulmonary vascular changes following mitral valvuloplasty. An anatomic and physiologic study. Am J Med 1968; 45:975–82.
8. Roy SB, Bhatia ML, Lazaro EJ, Ramalingaswami V. Juvenile mitral stenosis in India. Lancet 1963; 2:1193–5.
9. Tandon HD, Kasturi J. Pulmonary vascular changes associated with isolated mitral stenosis in India. Br Heart J 1975; 37:26–36.
10. Ferencz C. Pulmonary vascular changes in tetralogy of Fallot. Dis Chest 1964; 46:664–70.
11. Wagenvoort CA, Edwards JE. The pulmonary arterial tree in pulmonic atresia. Arch Pathol 1961; 71:646–53.

3. The adolescent and adult with complex congenital heart disease: which patients should we offer surgery?

DOUGLAS D. MAIR

Of more than 400 patients with congenital heart disease presenting to the Mayo Clinic annually to be evaluated for potential surgical intervention, approximately 25 percent are adolescents or adults. These patients, many of whom have been subjected to longstanding arterial hypoxemia and ventricular volume overloading, present special challenges in determining whether surgery can be expected to improve their quality and quantity of life, as contrasted to the natural history of their clinical course without additional operation. The two groups of such patients on whom this paper will focus are those with tricuspid atresia and Ebstein's anomaly.

Tricuspid atresia

Of the more than 800 Fontan procedures which have been performed at the Mayo Clinic since 1973 for patients with functional single ventricle, the largest anatomic subgroup of patients are those with tricuspid atresia. From 1973 to March 1989, 176 patients with tricuspid atresia had the Fontan procedure performed at the Mayo Clinic. During the initial eight-year experience from 1973 through 1980 there were 54 operations, whereas during the more recent approximate eight-year interval from 1981 to March 1989 there were 122. One hundred fifty-one patients had normally related great arteries and in 25 patients the great arteries were transposed. None of the 25 transposed great artery patients had significant subaortic obstruction pre-operatively.

Ages at operation, ranging from 7 months to 42 years, are listed in Table 1. It can be seen that a significant proportion of these patients were adolescents or adults with 43 patients, or nearly one-fourth of the group, being beyond the maximum age of 15 years proposed in the original criteria for operability established by Choussat and Fontan.

John Hess and George R. Sutherland (eds.), Congenital Heart Disease in Adolescents and Adults, 35–49.
© 1992 Kluwer Academic Publishers. Printed in the Netherlands.

Table 1. Age at operation.

Age at operation (yr)	Patients (n)
<2	3
2–3	20
4–6	40
7–10	37
11–15	33
16–19	20
20–30	16
31–40	6
>40	1
Total	176

Table 2. Previous palliative operations.

Previous cardiovascular surgical procedures	Patients (n)
0	15
1	105
2	45
3	11
Total	176

Only 15 patients had undergone no previous cardiovascular palliation prior to the Fontan procedure (Table 2). One hundred five patients had undergone one palliative procedure, 45 patients two palliative operations, and 11 patients three attempts at palliation.

The types of prior palliation are listed in Table 3. A standard or modified Blalock-Taussig anastomosis was the most frequently employed shunt followed by the Waterston, Glenn, and Potts anastomosis. Twenty-three patients had

Table 3. Types of palliation.

Types of previous palliative procedure	Procedures (n)
Blalock-Taussig (standard or modified)	107
Waterston	40
Glenn	33
Pulmonary artery banding	23
Potts	15
Blalock-Hanlon	5
Other	5
Total	228

undergone pulmonary artery banding, the majority of those being from the patient group with transposition of the great arteries.

Modifications in surgical techniques for the Fontan procedure have evolved significantly with experience. Five patients, all operated upon before 1978, had a porcine gluteraldehyde-preserved heterograft valve placed at the inferior vena cava-to-right atrial junction. However, this approach was abandoned when it was learned that these valves degenerated and became nonfunctional and obstructive. The type of connection used to direct systemic venous blood to the pulmonary arteries in these patients is given in Table 4. The use of valved conduits was also characteristic of the early experience, with all four of the right atrial to pulmonary artery valved conduits and 16 of the 26 right atrium-to-right ventricle valved conduits being placed before 1980. In the early years, an attempt was often made to incorporate the hypoplastic right ventricle into the circulation in patients with normally related great arteries, using either a right atrial-to-hypoplastic right ventricle pericardial patch or conduit. More recently, however, the method of choice for directing systemic venous blood to the pulmonary arteries has been direct anastomosis of the right atrium or right atrial appendage to the right or main pulmonary artery. This is reflected in the fact that in a previous report on the initial 90 patients of this series, 43 (48%) had a right atrium-to-right ventricle connection, whereas this approach has been used in only 18 of the 86 patients (21%) subsequently operated on in the past five years. Presently, the right ventricle is incorporated only when it is unusually well developed, being at least one third the normal expected volume; when this connection is made, a homograft contaning a valve is used to establish the right atrial-to-right ventricular communication.

Table 4. Types of connection.

Type of connection	Patients (n)
Right atrium-to-pulmonary artery direct anastomosis	111
Right atrium-to-pulmonary artery valved conduit	4
Right atrium-to-right ventricle anastomosis	35
Right atrium-to-right ventricle valved conduit	26
Total	176

Additional procedures carried out at the time of the Fontan procedure included mitral annuloplasty in four patients and mitral valve replacement in six patients, all of whom had moderate to severe mitral valve incompetence. In three of the valve replacements, a heterograft valve (Hancock) was used; in the other three a mechanical valve was inserted. Twenty patients had varying degrees of pulmonary artery reconstruction carried out, usually to alleviate narrowing and distortion caused by a prior shunt; the Waterston and Potts shunts being those most often causing this complicating feature. Two patients, one with a prior Waterston shunt and one with a prior Potts shunt performed during early infancy, had complete occlusion of the left pulmonary artery with some secondary hyperplasia of the right pulmonary artery; in those cases the Fontan procedure was performed to the single right pulmonary artery.

In the postoperative Fontan patient with normal central pulmonary arteries, the right-sided pressures are primarily dependent on pulmonary arteriolar resistance (Rp_a) and left ventricular diastolic compliance, the two resistances then in series.

Rp_a is determined at preoperative catheterization by dividing the mean driving pressure across the lungs (mean pulmonary artery pressure minus mean left atrial pressure) by the pulmonary flow index as determined by Fick oximetric method. An estimate of ventricular diastolic compliance may be obtained by dividing the ventricular end-diastolic pressure by the total volume load to which the ventricle is being subjected. In patients with tricuspid atresia, the left ventricle is receiving blood from and pumping blood to both the pulmonary and systemic circulations. The total volume load on the ventricle, therefore, is the pulmonary flow index plus the systemic flow index (Qp_I plus Qs_I), and the estimate of ventricular compliance is left ventricular end-diastolic pressure divided by Qp_I plus Qs_I. We retrospectively correlated postoperative right-sided pressures and clinical results with a new preoperative catheterization index obtained by adding Rp_a to left ventricular end-diastolic pressure divided by Qp_I plus Qs_I; the results from this analysis will be presented.

Results

Hospital, late, and overall mortality rates for patients operated on during the approximate eight-year intervals from 1973 through 1980 and 1981 through March 1989 are given in Table 5. It can be seen that operative mortality has been reduced to 8% during the most recent interval. Neither early nor overall mortality had a strongly significant relationship to age at the time of operation.

Causes of late death included reoperation, sudden death secondary to a presumed dysrhythmia, thromboembolism, progressive myocardial failure, and protein-losing enteropathy. One additional patient was killed when riding in an automobile involved in an accident.

Table 5. Operative results.

Year of operation	Patients (n)	Deaths (n)		Deaths (%)	
		Early	Late	Early	Overall
1973–1980	54	9	7	17[a]	30
1981–1989	122	10	3	8[a]	11
Total	176	19	10[b]		

[a]Not significant by χ^2.
[b]Excludes one patient killed as passenger in automobile accident.

Four of six patients having mitral replacement at the time of the Fontan procedure survived operation and continue to do well. Both patients with a single right pulmonary artery survived; one has had an excellent result, but the other is classified as fair.

A total of 19 reoperations were necessary in 17 patients. Reasons for reoperation included conduit replacement (4 patients), conduit removal and establishment of direct right atrium-to-pulmonary artery anastomosis (3 patients) pacemaker insertion (3 patients), and recurrent atrial septal defect (2 patients). Other complications (requiring reoperation in one patient each) included conduit removal and mitral valve replacement, pacemaker insertion and mitral valve replacement, enlargement of the right atrium-to-pulmonary artery anastomosis, takedown of the right atrium-to-right ventricular anastomosis and establishment of a direct right atrium to pulmonary artery anastomosis, left pulmonary artery patch enlargement, insertion of a right atrial to right ventricular homograft, and resection of severe aortic stenosis. Two patients died at the time of reoperation and two others survived reoperation but subsequently were late deaths secondary to a sudden dysrhythmia in one instance and progressive left ventricular failure in the other.

We have retrospectively assessed the preoperative catheterization data in our group of patients and correlated the new index, derived by adding Rp_a to left ventricular end-diastolic pressure divided by Qp_l plus Qs_l, the two resistances in series after completion of the procedure, to right-sided pressures measured intraoperatively after repair and to operative results. All patients with significant central pulmonary artery hypoplasia or distortion were eliminated from the review, as were patients with more than mild mitral valve incompetence, a factor that would increase left ventricular volume load in a manner that could not be accurately quantitated. Patients with a prior Glenn anastomosis in whom Rp_a could not be calculated were eliminated as were patients with unequal pressures in the right and left pulmonary arteries secondary to a Waterston or Potts shunt or secondary to a pulmonary artery banding impinging unequally on the two pulmonary arteries. In some patients, the preoperative catheterization data were incomplete (e.g. no pulmonary artery pressure, no systemic flow index), and the patients could not be included.

Sixty-eight patients were found to be acceptable candidates for this analysis. Table 6 gives a comparison of early and overall mortality rates with the preoperative catheterization index. It is seen that once this index exceeds 3.0, operative and overall mortality rates increase; once the index exceeds 4.0, this mortality increase is very substantial.

Intraoperative postrepair right atrial mean pressure was recorded in 171 of 176 patients (Table 7). This pressure is measured with the patient off cardiopulmonary bypass at a time when he or she is generating a systemic arterial pressure adequate to provide good peripheral perfusion. It can be seen that in patients in whom this mean right atrial pressure exceeds 20 mmHg, early and overall mortality rates increase very significantly.

Table 6. Preoperative chatheterization index and operative results.

Index[a]	Patients (n)	Deaths (n)		Deaths (%)	
		Early	Late	Early	Overall
<1.0	0	–	–	–	–
1.1–2.0	19	1	0	5 ⎫	5 ⎫
2.1–3.0	17	1	0	6 ⎬ 8[b]	6 ⎬ 8
3.1–4.0	14	2	0	14 ⎭	14 ⎭
4.1–5.0	11	·2	1	18 ⎫ 28[b]	27 ⎫ 39
>5.0	7	3	1	43 ⎭	57 ⎭
Total	68	9	2		

[a]Rp_a units $m^2 + \dfrac{LVEDP}{Qp_l + Qs_l}$.

[b]$p < 0.025$ by Wilcoxon rank-sum.

Table 7. Intraoperative postrepair right atrial mean pressure and operative results.

Postrepair right atrial mean pressure (mmHg)	Patients (n)	Deaths (n)		Deaths (%)	
		Early	Late	Early	Overall
⩽10	7	0	0	0 ⎫	0 ⎫
11–15	34	2	2	6 ⎬ 5[a]	12 ⎬ 11
16–20	108	6	6	6 ⎭	11 ⎭
21–25	20	9	1	45 ⎫ 45[a]	50 ⎫ 55
>25	2	1	1	50 ⎭	100 ⎭
Total	171[b]	18	10		

[a]$p < 0.001$ by Wilcoxon rank-sum.
[b]Not available in five patients.

Table 8 gives the comparison of intraoperative postrepair right atrial mean pressure with the preoperative catheterization index. In 60 patients in whom this index was available, the right atrial mean pressure was 20 mmHg or less. In this group the mean value of the catheterization index was 2.6 (range 1.1–5.1). Eight patients had a right atrial mean pressure of more than 20 mmHg; for this

Table 8. Intraoperative postrepair right atrial mean pressure versus preoperative catheterization index.

Postoperative right atrial mean pressure (mmHg)	Patients (n)	Index	
		Mean	Range
⩽20[a]	60	2.6[c]	1.1–5.1
⩾20[b]	8	4.7[c]	4.0–5.3

[a]Early mortality rate, 5%.
[b]Early mortality rate, 45%.
[c]$p < 0.001$ by Wilcoxon rank-sum.

group the mean catheterization index was 4.7 (range 4.0–5.3). It should be noted that no patient with a postoperative right atrial mean pressure of more than 20 mmHg, a group characterized by 45% early and 55% overall mortality rates, had a preoperative catheterization index of less than 4.0. Thus in our experience if this index, which incorporates both preoperative Rp_a and left ventricular diastolic function, is less than 4.0, right atrial mean pressure can be expected to be 20 mmHg or less after repair, a circumstance associated with 5% early and 11% overall mortality rates in the 171 patients in our series in whom this postrepair pressure was recorded.

Recent follow-up ($\leqslant 1$ year) from the patient or the patient's parent, if appropriate, was available for 139 patients (mean 5.5 years; maximum 14 years). Ninety-one percent of the patients were classified as being in excellent or good condition, and 9% were classified as being in fair or poor condition. Fifty-eight percent were receiving no cardiovascular medication, and most felt that they had a distinctly improved exercise tolerance compared with their preoperative status. One woman has delivered a normal infant after an uncomplicated pregnancy and delivery. In patients with a fair or poor result, complaints were primarily those of poor stamina and/or fluid retention with periodic pleural effusion, ascites, and so on. Two patients are known to have significant protein-losing enteropathy.

Discussion

Choussat and Fontan [1] originally listed ten criteria that they felt must be fulfilled before this procedure could be performed. With experience, it has become clear that this initial list was too stringent and that excellent results could be obtained in patients not satisfying one or more of these original criteria [2]. Many patients have done well when operated upon before the recommended minimum age of 4 years [3] or after the recommended maximum age of 15 years [4]. Absence of normal sinus rhythm preoperatively is not a contraindication [5] and anomalies of systemic and pulmonary venous return, common in the asplenia and polysplenia syndromes, can be handled well by the innovative surgeon [6]. Significant mitral valve incompetence, although it mandates concomitant valve repair or replacement at the time of the Fontan operation, does not in itself preclude the procedure if ventricular function remains good. It has become clear that the important criteria that must be satisfied to obtain a good operative result involve the central pulmonary arteries, pulmonary arterioles, and ventricular function, particularly diastolic compliance. The maintenance of a satisfactory cardiac output at acceptably low right-sided pressures in the postoperative Fontan patient mandates that there be relatively unimpeded flow through the central pulmonary arteries and pulmonary resistance vessels. In addition, the filling pressure of the left ventricle must be low enough so that when the 6–8 mmHg mean transpulmonary gradient that is necessary under the best of circumstances to drive blood across the pulmonary capillary bed is added to the mean left-sided filling pressures, there is not a resulting mean pressure in the right atrium and systemic veins of more than 18–20 mmHg.

The central pulmonary arteries in most patients with functional single ventricles are not naturally hypoplastic; if problems with these vessels are present they are most often iatrogenic, secondary to distortion from a previous shunt or a pulmonary artery band. The Waterston and Potts shunts are particularly prone to scar and produce hypoplasia of the central pulmonary arteries; in this era, these shunts should be avoided in favor of the less mutilating Blalock-Taussig shunt or an aorta-to-pulmonary artery Goretex graft.

A large series from another institution [3] revealed a significantly increased operative mortality rate if Rp_a exceeded 2.0 units m^2, and our experience has been similar with patients in whom Rp_a was more than 3.0 units m^2 [2].

Ventricular diastolic function is often difficult to assess at preoperative catheterization in these patients who often have ventricular volume loads of threefold or more that of normal with equally increased ventricular dimensions. Postoperatively, once the ventricular volume load has been reduced to normal, the ventricular end-diastolic pressure of no more than 12 to 14 mmHg is mandatory if right-sided pressures are to be acceptably low. Many of these patients, however, have a ventricular end-diastolic pressure of 15–20 mmHg or more before the Fontan operation, and it is necessary to determine whether this elevated pressure is secondary to the increased ventricular volume load and hence can be expected to decrease significantly immediately after surgery or whether it is largely due to ventricular hypertrophy and fibrosis and therefore will not decrease significantly after the procedure. An elevated left ventricular end-diastolic pressure divided by a large volume load may indicate a normal compliance that will manifest itself in an acceptably low left ventricular end-diastolic pressure immediately postoperatively when the ventricular volume load has been normalized. However, an elevated left ventricular end-diastolic pressure divided by a relatively modest ventricular volume load will give a higher value that may indicate reduced myocardial compliance, in which case the immediate postoperative left-sided pressures may remain significantly elevated and preclude an operative survivor or a good result.

In reviewing our results it appears clear that if the new preoperative catheterization index that we have proposed exceeds 4.0, then the risk of surgery increases significantly. However, a value of more than 4.0 does not conclusively indicate that the patient is a poor operative risk. Two of our patients who postoperatively had a right atrial mean pressure of 20 mmHg or less had preoperative catheterization indexes of 4.9 and 5.1. These patients' (each was <3 years old) elevated values were due to an Rp_a on room air of 3.7 and 4.0 units m^2, respectively. Therefore, the elevated preoperative catheterization indexes in these two pateints were manifestations of high Rp_a on room air rather than of a problem with ventricular diastolic compliance. Each patient had an elevated mean pulmonary artery pressure of approximately 30 mmHg in the presence of a large pulmonary blood flow. When they were given 100% oxygen to breath in the cardiac catheterization laboratory, Rp_a decreased to 1.7 and 1.9 units m^2, respectively. If these values had been added to the left ventricular diastolic compliance values, preoperative catheterization indexes would have been well below 4.0. In patients with elevated pulmonary artery pressure and large pulmonary blood flow, there is often an element of pulmonary arteriolar vasoconstriction on room air that increases Rp_a. Such patients should always be placed on 100% oxygen breathing in the cardiac laboratory; if their Rp_a and hence their preoperative catheterization index decreases appreciably, they may well prove to be good surgical candidates. If, however, Rp_a and catheterization index remain high while the patients breath 100% oxygen, such patients will clearly be in the high risk operative group.

Our extensive experience to date with the Fontan approach for tricuspid atresia has in general been most rewarding. The operative risk, is now less than 10% and the majority of operative survivors are doing well. Most patients or parents of patients report a subjective improvement in exercise tolerance compared with preoperative conditions, and there is objective evidence as well that this occurs [7].

Truly long term results from the Fontan operation remain to be determined with the majority of our patients still less than ten years postoperative. Will there be late problems secondary to nonpulsatile pulmonary flow or systemic venous hypertension? To date we have not seen pulmonary arteriovenous fistulae develop in our postoperative Fontan patients, a complication which has been seen in patients with longstanding Glenn anastomoses. Liver function tests in patients returning postoperatively have been normal with no patient having significant liver dysfunction to date. Protein-losing enteropathy [8] is a complication which has been seen in approximately 2.5 percent of our Fontan population. In some patients this can be managed using combinations of medical therapy and diet but in some patients it has been quite refractory to treatment, resulting in either death or a poor late result. Significant atrial dysrhythmias have been seen in approximately 7 percent of our postoperative Fontan patients, some of whom also had an atrial dysrhythmia preoperatively. These dysrhythmias can usually be managed medically although some have proved quite troublesome and on occasion necessitated the implantation of an antitachycardia pacemaker. Thromboembolic phenomena, [9] though not common, have been observed in our postoperative tricuspid atresia patients and were responsible for three late deaths in this group. A small percentage of our post-Fontan patients have had laminated thrombus echocardiographically visible in the right atrium without clinical sequelae to date. The question of anticoagulating postoperative Fontan patients, and if so for how long, remains controversial but to date we have not routinely anticoagulated these patients. The ability for the postoperative Fontan adult female to withstand pregnancy is a question which is being asked with increasing frequency as these patients reach the childbearing age. Clearly pregnancy must carry some increased risk, both to the mother and to the fetus, in this group of patients but it would appear that in patients who have had a good hemodynamic result that pregnancy and delivery can be tolerated and pregnancy probably should not be discouraged in such patients if they strongly desire a family.

The results of the Fontan operation in patients with tricuspid atresia have in general been gratifying. Follow-up reveals subjective and objective evidence of significantly improved quality of life in the majority of cases. Although late complications are seen in some patients, it seems likely that with continued surgical and medical innovations, and early operative intervention, that their incidence will decrease. Clearly additional years must pass before firm conclusions can be drawn about the success of this operative approach but the initial nearly two decades of experience strongly suggest that it represents a major step forward in providing help and hope to a group of patients afflicted with one of the most complex forms of congenital heart disease. We now feel quite comfortable in recommending the Fontan operation to properly selected patients and experience has proven [4] that a significant proportion of adolescents and adults who remain excellent candidates will benefit from this operative approach.

Ebstein's anomaly

We shall now turn our attention to Ebstein's anomaly. There is probably no congenital heart lesion in which the spectrum of clinical symptomatology can vary over a greater age range than with this lesion. Severe forms of the malformation may result in intrauterine death or death within the very early neonatal period in the live born infant. On the other end of the spectrum an autopsy-documented case of this condition seen at the Mayo Clinic had no cardiovascular symptoms until the age of 79 and lived to the age of 85, dying of a malignancy. Clearly most patients with this deformity lie between these two extremes insofar as symptomatology is concerned but there is no question that many patients will remain essentially symptom free until adolescence or early adulthood. Once clinical deterioration does begin, however, the downhill course may be very rapid and patients who are severely symptomatic with massive cardiac enlargement may, in some instances, have lost their best chance for significant help brought about by surgical intervention.

Clinical symptoms in patients with Ebstein's malformation are caused by alterations in hemodynamics, or disorders of cardiac rhythm, or both. Hemodynamic alterations are most common secondary to tricuspid insufficiency, although in rare cases tricuspid stenosis may be present. In addition, the frequently associated atrial septal defect often results in significant right-to-left shunting, secondary hypoxemia, and polycythemia, which can be of a severe degree. Pulmonary stenosis may also be present and accentuate the degree of tricuspid insufficiency, or right-to-left shunting, or both.

The incidence of clinically significant rhythm disorders in patients with Ebstein's malformation is approximately 20 percent in most large series of reported cases. Paroxysmal supraventricular tachycardia is by far the most frequent rhythmic disorder. It often is the result of an accessory conduction pathway (the Wolff-Parkinson-White syndrome) that produces pre-excitation and which can also result in a re-entrant tachycardia. Medical management of a clinically significant recurrent tachycardia is always tried initially. If it is unsuccessful and the patient has an accessory conduction pathway, surgical division of the pathway should be considered; this approach has produced a large measure of success in recent years.

Early attempts at surgical correction of Ebstein's malformation involved replacement of the tricuspid valve with a prosthetic valve; these attempts were generally unsuccessful. More recently, a new surgical approach utilizing plastic reconstruction of the patient's natural valve has evolved and has produced better results [10]. The surgical technique, applicable in 75 percent of patients, involves plication of the free wall of the right ventricle, posterior tricuspid annuloplasty, and reduction in the size of the right atrium. Any associated defect (atrial septal defect or pulmonary stenosis, among others) is also corrected at the time of the tricuspid valve repair. The operation is based on the principle of establishing a competent monocusp valve by using the anterior leaflet of the tricuspid valve, which is usually large in this condition. For the repair to succeed, the anterior leaflet must be of sufficient size and the free edge cannot be tethered to the endocardial surface of the heart. In experienced hands, two-dimensional echocardiography has been a highly reliable method of ascertaining the anatomy of the tricuspid valve in Ebstein's malformation patients and of determining if the anterior leaflet will lend itself to a plastic reconstruction of the valve [11, 12].

Between 1972 and March 1987, the last time follow-up was undertaken, 122 patients with Ebstein's had undergone surgery at the Mayo Clinic. Through March of 1990 this series had increased in size to 158 patients. All operated patients were either significantly symptomatic or were demonstrating rapidly progressive increase in heart size. In the series through March 1987 (Table 9), 90, or approximately 75 percent, had valve reconstruction. Twenty-eight patients had required insertion of a bioprosthesis and in four a Fontan procedure was performed because of a severely thinned out and noncontractile right ventricle. There were six early deaths, an operative mortality of 4.9 percent, and all occurred in severely symptomatic patients in whom the cardiothoracic ratio preoperatively exceeded 0.65.

Table 9. Surgical repair of Ebstein's anomaly.

Procedure	Patient (n)	Early deaths	
		No.	%
Plication and annuloplasty	90	5	5.6
Pliation and bioprosthesis	28	1	3.5
Plication and Fontan	4	0	0
Total	122	6	4.9

Age distribution at operation is illustrated in Table 10. Fifty-two patients, or 43 percent, were age 20 or greater and 71, or 58 percent, were age 16 or greater.

Associated procedures at the time of operation are shown in Table 11. One hundred six patients had concomitant closure of an atrial septal defect. In 16 patients an accessory conduction pathway characteristic of the Wolff-Parkinson-White syndrome was divided and in all instances this division was successful, with no postoperative return of pre-excitation or supraventricular tachycardia.

Table 10. Age distribution of Ebstein's anomaly.

Age	Patient (n)
11–23 months	7
2–9 years	21
10–19 years	42
20–29 years	33
30–64 years	19
Total	122

Table 11. Associated procedures in Ebstein's anomaly.

Procedure	Patient (n)
Repair ASD	106
Division accessory pathway	16
Repair pulmonary stenosis	12
Closure shunt	6
Repair parital anomalous pulmonary venous connection	2
Repair VSD	3
Closure RA-LA fistula	1
Pericardiectomy	1

At the time of most recent follow-up in 1987 subjective exercise tolerance data were obtained from 44 patients, ranging from 1 to 14 years postoperatively. Thirty-nine (85%) of these patients were in New York Heart Association Class I or II. Three patients were in Class III and there were two late deaths. Both late deaths were sudden and unexpected and were presumed due to a ventricular dysrhythmia. Five women have undergone successful preganancy and delivery. In patients reassessed by cardiac catheterization, or two-dimensional echocardiography, or both, efficient tricuspid valve function was minimal or no incompetence has been documented.

Based upon the surgical experience previously described, we now believe that in patients beyond early infancy and significantly symptomatic because of tricuspid valve dysfunction or hypoxemia secondary to right-to-left atrial-level shunting, surgical intervention should be carried out. In approximately 75 percent of these patients adequate valve reconstruction will be possible. In 25 percent the anatomy of the anterior leaflet may preclude a plastic repair, and valve replacement may be necessary. In patients needing valve replacement, particularly if the initial operation occurs in early childhood, reoperation for insertion of a new valve eventually may be necessary. If this is the case, the risk of reoperation should be low and the eventual result satisfactory. The risk of operation in patients with Ebstein's malformation is relatively low. Because the natural history of the deformity has been established to be very poor, once patients become significantly symptomatic, this aggressive surgical approach seems to be justifiable.

Since the advent of two-dimensional echocardiography, we have found that preoperative cardiac catheterization is rarely necessary in patients with Ebstein's malformation. Two-dimensional echocardiography can establish the diagnosis conclusively [11, 12], including the presence of associated lesions, such as an atrial septal defect or pulmonary stenosis. This modality shows the anatomy of the tricuspid valve more precisely than does angiocardiography and can accurately predict if plastic reconstruction of the tricuspid valve is feasible or valve replacement is likely to be necessary. Only if the significance of an associated lesion, such as pulmonary stenosis or ventricular septal defect was in question, would we now recommend preoperative catheterization.

A question arises as to whether patients who remain in New York Heart Association Class I or II should have 'elective' repair of their Ebstein's deformity carried out because of the manifestations of progressive significant cardiomegaly, a paradoxic embolus, or significant hypoxemia and polycythemia. In the follow-up of the Mayo Clinic surgical series, it was apparent that the few patients who had less satisfactory late results and who still had significant exercise intolerance or problems with ventricular dysrhythmias after operation were those in whom severe cardiomegaly (cardiothoracic ratio >0.65) was present before operation. This being the case and with the operation now being well established as effective therapy that can be accomplished at relatively low risk, we favor elective operative intervention in patients with significant progression in heart size. The operation should be carried out before the cardiothoracic ratio exceeds 0.65. This decision is made easier if two-dimensional echocardiography indicates that plastic repair of the valve, rather than valve replacement, is feasible.

The question of whether to recommend 'elective' operation to prevent or to eliminate the physiologic consequences of the right-to-left atrial level shunt in patients who continue to do well is more difficult to answer. If surgical therapy is to be offered under such circumstances, should it be merely closure of the atrial septal defect or should the tricuspid valve also be repaired? Based upon the operative and late results obtained at this Institution over the past decade, we now think it wise to recommend operation for patients who have had a significant embolic event or in whom there is clinically significant cyanosis or polycythemia. If operation is to be carried out in these patients, we deem it appropriate to perform both reconstruction of the tricuspid valve and closure of the atrial septal defect. The decision-making in these cases is again made easier if plastic valve reconstruction appears to be feasible on the basis of preoperative echocardiographic evaluation.

Finally, on occasion the surgeon may be called upon to divide an accessory conduction pathway that is precipitating bouts of supraventricular tachycardia, which are poorly controlled medically, in a patient with Ebstein's malformation in whom the hemodynamic alternations secondary to the deformity appear to be mild. Under these circumstances, should the surgeon also attempt to repair the tricuspid valve and close the atrial septal defect if one is present? Closure of an atrial septal defect or patent foramen ovale can be accomplished so rapidly and with so little risk of complication that it clearly seems reasonable. Whether to intervene surgically on a valve, which although malformed is not significantly incompetent, is more problematic. However, in many patients the degree of incompetence will gradually worsen with time. Encouraged by the operative results to date, we now think that valve repair snould be carried out under these special circumstances.

The current low operative mortality, the fact that a plastic repair is feasible in the majority of cases, and the encouraging follow-up results all lead us to believe that surgical treatment is now advisable for all patients with Ebstein's malformation who, despite medical therapy, have deteriorated into New York Heart Association class III or beyond. We now also recommend operation for patients who are less symptomatic but who exhibit progressive significant cardiomegaly, hypoxemia, or polycythemia, or who have suffered a paradoxic embolus. The ability to predict, through two-dimensional echocardiography, those patients who will be candidates for valvuloplasty and those who will probably need valve replacement, assists in the decision-making, in borderline situations.

References

1. Choussat A, Fontan F, Besse P, Vallot F, Chauve A, Bricaud H. Selection criteria for Fontan procedure. In: Anderson RH, Shinbourne EA, editors. Pediatric cardiology. Edinburgh: Churchill Livingstone, 1978:559–66.
2. Mair DD, Rice MJ, Hagler DJ, Puga FJ, McGoon DC, Danielson GK. Outcome of the Fontan procedure in patients with tricuspid atresia. Circulation 1985:72(Suppl II):II–88–II–92.
3. Mayer JE, Helgason H, Jonas RA, et al. Extending the limits for modified Fontan precedures. J. Thorac Cardiovasc Surg 1986;92:1021–8.
4. Humes RA, Mair DD, Porter CJ, Puga FJ, Schaff HV, Danielson GK. Results of the modified Fontan operation in adults. Am J Cardiol 1988;61:602–4.
5. Albolaris ET, Porter CJ, Danielson GK et al. Results of the modified Fontan operation for congenital heart lesions in patients without preoperative sinus rhythm. Am J Cardiol 1985;6:228–33.
6. Humes RA, Feldt RH, Porter CJ, Julsrud PA, Puga FJ, Danielson GK. The modified Fontan operation for asplenia and polysplenia syndromes. J Thorac Cardiovasc Surg 1988;96:212–8.
7. Driscoll DJ, Danielson GK, Puga FJ, Schaff HV, Heise CT, Staats BA. Exercise tolerance and cardiorespiratory response to exercise after the Fontan operation for tricuspid atresia of functional single ventricle. J Am Coll Cardiol 1986;7:1087–94.

8. Crupi G, Locatelli G, Tiraboschi R, Villani M, Detommasi M, Parenzan L. Protein-losing enteropathy after Fontan operation for tricuspid atresia (imperforate tricuspid valve). Thorac Cardiovasc Surg 1980;28:359–63.

9. Shannon FL, Campbell DN, Clarke DR. Right atrial thrombosis: Rare complication of the modified Fontan. Pediatr Cardiol 1986;7:209–12.

10. Danielson GK, Maloney JD, Devloo RAE. Surgical Repair of Ebstein's Anomaly. Mayo Clinic Proc 1979;54:185.

11. Shina A, Seward JB, Edwards WD, Hagler DJ, Tajik AJ. Two-dimensional echocardiographic spectrum of Ebstein's anomaly: Detailed anatomic assessment. J Am Coll Cardiol 1984;3(2):356–70.

12. Shina A, Seward JB, Tajik AJ, Hagler DJ, Danielson GK. Two-dimensional echocardiographic-surgical correlation in Ebstein's anomaly: Preoperative determination of patients requiring tricuspid valve plication versus replacement. Circulation 1983;68(3):534–44.

4. Transoesophageal echocardiography in adolescents and adults with congenital heart disease

GEORGE R. SUTHERLAND & OLIVER F.W. STÜMPER

Introduction

The number of patients with complex congital heart disease who are surviving into adult life is rapidly increasing. This is a direct result of the improvements in cardiac surgery in the 1970s and 80s. The majority of such patients will have undergone complex corrective operations. Many will have important residual cardiac abnormalities. Such lesions may remain unchanged in the post-operative period; others may develop or progress in the early or late post-operative period. Until the introduction of cardiac ultrasound, the detailed investigation of such patients relied on the acquisition of invasive data at cardiac catheterisation. In recent years with the introduction of high resolution 2-D imaging of the heart allied to the definition of intra cardiac flow patterns by colour flow mapping and the evaluation of intra cardiac pressure drops by spectral doppler, much of the information previously available from cardiac catheterisation is now available from detailed cardiac ultrasound studies. In virtually all unoperated infants and children, ultrasound can be used with great accuracy to establish the correct morphologic diagnosis and to define the consequent haemodynamics. This information alone can be used to plan the requirement for surgical intervention [1]. However the problems faced following corrective or palliative surgery are different. These older children, who have a natural reduction in their praecordial ultrasound window with age, normally have a further reduction or obliteration of this window following sternotomy or thoracotomy. This significantly reduces the number of post operative patients in whom a full cardiac ultrasound examination can be carried out from the praecordium. This problem is much worse in the adult age group. Other non-invasive diagnostic techniques have been tried as alternative methods of non-invasive assessment in these complex patients. Both Computed Tomography and Magnetic Resonance Imaging have been advocated as alternative diagnostic approaches. The former has found little favour in this

John Hess and George R. Sutherland (eds.), Congenital Heart Disease in Adolescents and Adults, 51–78.
© 1992 *Kluwer Academic Publishers. Printed in the Netherlands.*

patient group but Magnetic Resonnance Imaging (MRI) has found a number of proponents. MRI however remains in its infancy and as currently formatted cannot supply the range of information which the cardiologist requires. It is seen at its most valuable in the assessment of the morphology of the thoracic aorta and the central pulmonary arteries and at present that would appear to be its most valuable application in the assessment of complex heart disease. Since the introduction of high resolution transoesophageal echocardiographic imaging (incorporating colour flow mapping and spectral doppler modalities) an alternative diagnostic approach, albeit not strictly non-invasive has become available for use in the diagnosis and follow-up of these patients.

It is the aim of this article to attempt to define the current role of transoesophageal imaging in adults with congenital heart disease. The conclusions that will be drawn about the current main indications for a transoesophageal study in adolescent and adult patients with congenital heart disease (Table 1) are based on experience gained in carrying out such studies in some 457 patients who have attended the Adolescent and Adult Congenital Heart Disease Clinics of either the Thoraxcentrum (Rotterdam) or the Royal Infirmary, Edinburgh. This work has, in part, already appeared in print [2].

Table. 1. The current main indications for transoesophageal studies in adolescent and adult patients with congenital heart disease.

Primary diagnosis	anomalous systemic venous connections
	anomalous pulmonary venous connections
	juxtaposition of the atrial appendages
	atrial septal defects
	atrioventricular junction abnormalities
	left ventricular outflow tract obstruction
	coronary artery fistulae
Monitoring	
a. perioperative	surgical repair at atrial level
	atrioventricular valve repair/replacement
	Mustard/Senning procedure
	Fontan-type procedures
	continuous monitoring during early post op period
	diagnosis and management of early post op complications
b. interventional catheterization	guidance of balloon catheter position
	exclusion of immediate complications
	assessment of immediate haemodynamic results/changes
	dilatations of venous pathway obstructions
	device closure of atrial septal effects
Follow-up	Mustard/Senning procedures
	Fontan-type procedures
	atrioventricular valve repair/replacement
	suspected residual or acquired atrial lesions

The equipment and techniques used for transoesophageal studies in the adolescent/adult age groups

Adolescent and adult transoesophageal probes

Transverse plane imaging
The most widely used transoesophageal probes in adult cardiology are systems built on an endoscope that has a maximal shaft diameter of some 10–11 mm, and a total shaft length of some 110 cm. The steering facilities of these probes normally provide both anterior/posterior and right/left lateral tip angulation. The length of the flexible portion of these probes measures some 10 cm. The distance from the maximal point of angulation to the very tip of the endoscope is normally some 7 cm. The ultrasound transducer itself is embedded in the most distal rectangular segment of the probe. The length of the tip normally measures some 23 mm, the maximal height most often 12–13 mm and the maximal width some 14–15 mm. Thus, the maximal tip circumference $[2 \times (\text{height} + \text{width})]$ most often exceeds 52 mm. Modifications in transducer tip design include a rounding of the rectangular tip design. This appears to facilitate the swallowing of the probe by the awake patient.

The majority of current generation single-plane probes use an imaging frequency centred around 5 or 5.6 MHz and are comprised of a phased array transducer containing 64 elements. The ultrasound elements are mounted at the flexible tip so as to provide transverse plane images of the heart, i.e. their scan plane is at right angles to the shaft of the endoscope. Cross-sectional imaging, in combination with colour flow mapping and pulsed wave Doppler interrogation is provided on all currently available probes. Most recently continuous wave Doppler facilities have become available on selected phased array transoesophageal probes. In addition, one annular array mechanical system is available, that allows a dynamic shift in imaging frequency from 5 to 7.5 MHz in combination with both high pulse repetition frequency Doppler and continuous wave Doppler.

Biplane imaging
In 1989, Omoto and colleagues introduced the first biplane transoesophageal probe for use in adult patients. Current generation biplane probes have two separate ultrasound transducer element arrays mounted at the tip of the scope so as to provide both transverse axis and longitudinal axis images of the heart and the great vessels. Conventionally, the more distal transducer provides the standard transverse axis images. By switching a button on the ultrasound system the more proximal transducer is activated and generates longitudinal plane images. Subsequent attempts to use the same set of ultrasound crystals to generate both imaging planes (using a matrix array format) have met with limited success so far. Since the advantages of biplane transoesophageal imaging have become increasingly apparent over the last two years [6, 7], more manufacturers have turned to this technology. In fact, with miniaturisation in

transducer design it is now possible to construct biplane transoesophageal probes with two sets of 64 element channels, which have similar dimensions to the current standard 64 element single-plane probes.

Multiplane imaging

The ultimate goal in transoesophageal probe design, however, remains the construction of high resolution multiplane imaging probes. Such probes are currently under development [8]. In these probes, a 48 or 64 element phased array transducer is mounted on a circular footprint, which can be rotated from 0 degrees (transverse plane) through 90 degrees (longitudinal plane) to almost 180 degrees (reversed transverse plane). Such systems have many theoretical and practical advantages. Since in clinical practice lateral angulation of an endoscope within the oesophagus beyond 30 degrees is rarely possible without causing considerable discomfort to the patient, this multiplane approach can provide a number of additional imaging planes not normally available using standard biplane probes. A further advantage of this system is that all the required imaging planes can normally be obtained from the one transducer position within the oesophagus. Initial clinical studies have documented that, firstly, such a transducer design is feasible and, secondly, that several advantages are provided over biplane imaging alone [9]. These include 1) three dimensional reconstruction of cardiac anatomy; 2) a better insight into certain aspects of mitral valve morphology and function; and 3) a more detailed assessment of the atrial septum and the great arteries. To a large extent, this probe design liberates transoesophageal imaging from the constraints of a tomographic imaging technique. Structures can be followed and connected by unlimited rotation of the probe, in a manner comparable to precordial imaging.

Techniques

The physician who undertakes transoesophageal studies should either have a sound experience in gastroenterology or should be trained specifically to perform oesophageal intubation. It is our opinion that a sufficient experience can be acquired by observing some 20 gastroscopies and thereafter by performing another 20 to 40 esophageal intubations under supervision.

All patients who are scheduled for a transoesophageal echocardiographic study should have a history taken concerning current or previous upper gastrointestinal disease, spinal disease and bleeding disorders. The procedure should be explained in detail to the patient, as should be the reasons why such a study is undertaken. Written consent from the patients or their parents should be obtained. Patients should be fasted at least four hours prior to the procedure and any dental prosthesis should be removed.

Probe insertion

Prior to all studies the investigator should check on the proper function of the probe, both in terms of probe mechanics and transducer performance. The probe may then be inserted into a long plastic sheath, if that is the policy of the operator. The sheath should contain a sufficient amount of ultrasound gel at its tip. Care must be taken that there are no air bubbles left at the level of the transducer. As the sheath can cause discomfort to the patient, we and others, prefer to perform studies without the use of a sheath. In such cases, the shaft of the probe should be well lubricated. The probe must be carefully disinfected between studies.

Sterilization of the probe is carried out by thorough washing of the probe and by subsequent emersion in a Cidex solution for 20 minutes. Alcohol should not be used for disinfection since it may degrade the silicon material used to cover the ultrasound transducer. All transoesophageal probes should be routinely checked for electrical safety, as this may be compromised by the development of even microscopic cracks in the coating material.

Adolescents and adult studies in the outpatient clinic
The procedure should be explained to the patient in detail and reassurance given. Local anaesthesia (lidocaine spray) is applied to the hypo-pharynx and tongue, and the patient is then asked to swallow. Venous access should be established in all patients, and electrocardiographic leads connected to allow continuous ECG monitoring. Sedation should be used more liberally in adolescents and young adults with congenital heart disease, than in the older patient with acquired cardiac disease. This is, firstly, because transoesophageal studies in complex congenital heart disease tend to be more time consuming, and, secondly, patient tolerance towards oesophageal intubation is relatively poorer in the younger patient population. We currently prefer either Midazolam (3–5 mg) or Diazepam (5–8 mg) for sedation. Midazolam has the advantage of a more rapid and shorter action and better retrograde amnesia. In addition, its action can be reversed at the end of the pocedure. It is also our current practice to use a secretion-drying agent in all patients under the age of forty. This is because younger patients tend to produce copius secretions during the procedure. These may be intolerable to the patient resulting in the procedure having to be aborted. Our current preference is to use intravenous Glycopyrrelate in an appropriate dose per kilogram to reduce dry secretions.

The patient is then asked to roll over onto his or her left side and to approximate chin to chest. An absorbent drape is put under the patient's face and covering his shoulder and left arm. The bite guard is positioned over the shaft of the transoesophageal probe. The operator holds the handle of the probe with his left hand and the right hand supports the probe at a distance of roughly 20 cm from the tip. During insertion the tip of the transducer is initially flexed anteriorly so as to gain contact with the tongue. The probe is then gradually advanced until the hypopharynx is reached. Thereafter the tip of the probe is slightly retroflexed so as to gain contact with the posterior aspect of the hypopharynx and to stay away from the epiglottis. With the probe in this position the patient will normally gag. The patient is then asked to swallow and following successful swallowing the probe is then rapidly advanced in the oesophagus to the level of the left atrium. Probe advancement should never be carried out against resistance. Once the probe is inserted the patient is asked to breath normally and the biteguard is secured so as to prevent any damage of the transducer.

Certainly modifications of the above described technique of probe insertion exist, and individual operators will evolve their own methods of probe introduction with growing experience. However, despite the variations between individual techniques, several important aspects should be kept in mind. Firstly, the probe should always stay in a midline position during introduction in order to prevent passage into the (lateral) piriform recesses of the pharynx. Under no circumstances should the probe be advanced against resistance. Once the oesophagus has been entered, the probe should be advanced to a level well below the bifurcation of the trachea, where it causes the least discomfort to the patient. Both high oesophageal and gastric positions are less well tolerated.

Transoesophageal studies carried out under general anaesthesia

Transoesophageal studies performed in either the perioperative period or in the intensive care unit will normally be carried out with the patient under general anaesthesia using endotracheal intubation. With the patient in the supine position, it is best for the operator to introduce the probe and to perform the study standing at the patient's head. Nasogastric tubes should be removed prior to probe insertion. In our experience, it has proved easiest to place the probe and connecting cable around the operator's neck, and to introduce the distal portion of the probe into the hypopharynx with the right hand, while the left hand remains free for manipulation. During insertion, the left hand may be used to lift the patient's mandible and to slightly extent the patient's neck. In orally intubated patients, the partially flexed probe is then passed along the palate, above the endotracheal tube, and is advanced into the hypopharynx. In nasotracheally intubated patients in the intensive care unit, the probe should be inserted from a rather lateral position and is then passed behind the endotracheal tube into the oesophagus. In such cases the left index finger should be used for orientation and accurate probe guidance within the mouth. In cases in whom probe insertion fails or meets resistance, a further attempt may be undertaken and if this fails, the probe should then be inserted under direct laryngoscopic vision.

Monitoring

The combination of a reliable venous access and continuous electrocardiographic monitoring are prerequisites for all transoesophageal studies. In fact, such monitoring is sufficient for the majority of outpatient studies. In cyanotic patients the additional monitoring of oxygen saturations should be performed using a finger tip oximeter. Blood pressure monitoring in our experience is of little value in the outpatient setting. However, during studies in patients undergoing surgical correction or in the intensive care unit the echocardiographer should take advantage of the abundance of concomitant monitoring information available in these two clinical settings.

Transoesophageal studies in patients with congenital heart disease should only be performed in areas where there is equipment of cardiopulmonary resuscitation ready at hand. In particular, a reliable suction apparatus and oxygen supply are mandatory. A complete set of drugs for resuscitation should be prepared, and equipment for tracheal intubation and defibrillation should be available.

Endocarditis prophylaxis

In the past there has been evidence brought forward that bacteriemia is a frequent finding during transoesophageal studies. Thus, several investigators have advocated giving antibiotic endocarditis prophylaxis as a routine measure. This is in contrast to the experience with thousands of transoesophageal studies being performed without antibiotic prophylaxis with no case of associated endocarditis having been documented. Moreover, accepted guidelines on endocarditis prophylaxis do not list upper gastrointestinal diagnostic procedures as an indication. Recently, two prospective studies have reported on the incidence of positive blood cultures both during and after transoesophageal studies. These studies confirmed that the incidence of bacteraemia associated with gastroscopy is very low and may indeed be explained by contamination during blood sampling. We currently do not use antibiotic prophylaxis in any patient, and have not experienced a single case of endocarditis following a transoesophageal study in our extensive study population which has included both congenital (>650 cases) and acquired (>2500 cases) cardiac disease.

The standard examination protocol

Introduction

All transoesophageal studies carried out to assess congenital heart disease should follow a standardized scheme. The investigator should observe the rules of sequential chamber analysis, the approach most widely used in the categorization of congenital malformations of the heart. Firstly, the type of venous connections to the heart should be described. Thereafter the location and the morphology of the atrial chambers is assessed. Then the atrioventricular connection is defined and finally the form of the ventriculo-arterial connection is documented. Only thereafter are specific lesions more closely examined. This approach may appear time-consuming and complicated to the adult cardiologist, but it is only on the basis of this framework that the description of congenital cardiac malformations is meaningful.

The examination

The probe is initially advanced to image the transoesophageal four chamber plane. The position of the cardiac apex should be noted. This can be on the left, midline or on the patient's right side (dextrocardia). Minor degrees of cardiac malposition will go undetected by transoesophageal imaging. Patients with dextrocardia are as easily studied as normal patients. Probe manipulation in such cases just involves a ninety degree clockwise rotation of the probe from the normal oesophageal imaging position (whereas in precordial ultrasound techniques this requires a mirror image examination technique). After establishing the position of the cardiac apex, the probe should then be slightly advanced together with clockwise rotation of the probe, so as to demonstrate the liver from a scan position near the oesophageal hiatus. The infradiaphragmatic segment of the inferior caval vein is visualised by this manoeuvre and by gradual probe withdrawal, the pattern of drainage of the hepatic veins established. The distal portion of the inferior caval vein should then be followed to the (right) atrial chamber. Further probe withdrawal using right lateral scan positions will then demonstrate the connection of the superior caval vein to the atrial chamber. Immediately posterior to this the right upper pulmonary vein is visualised, and repeat probe insertion together with clockwise rotation will demonstrate the right lower pulmonary vein near its site of connection with the (left) atrial chamber. Ninety degree clockwise rotation of the probe will then allow visualization of the left lower pulmonary vein, and, following gradual probe withdrawal, the left upper pulmonary vein and their site of drainage to the atria. Colour flow mapping studies will help the rapid identification of the site of connections of the four pulmonary veins. The left sided atrial appendage is normally visualised just anterior and medially to the left upper pulmonary vein. The right atrial appendage should then be imaged by a clockwise rotation of the probe from this scan position. The examination of the morphologic features of either atrial appendage will then allow the direct diagnosis of the atrial arrangement. Following this documentation of the cardiac position, and the definition of both the venous connections and the atrial arrangement, the next step should be to define the type of atrioventricular connection using a series of transoesophageal four-chamber views. Finally the morphology of the ventriculo-aterial junction should be visualised by scanning high oesophageal views and the mode of ventriculo-arterial connection established. The relation of the great arteries to one another and to the underlying ventricular chambers is best defined using a series of slight probe manipulations.

Thus having defined the ventriculo-arterial connection and the spatial relations of the great vessels to one another, the process of sequential chamber localisation is complete and the transoesophageal examination should then proceed to the assessment of the individual lesions. This examination should also be performed in a standard sequential manner. The venous return to the heart should be assessed in more detail, as should be the atrial chambers, the atrial septum, the atrioventricular valves, the ventricular chambers and the ventricular septum and, finally, the great arteries. Colour flow mapping should be performed at all cardiac levels for the rapid identification of abnormal flow patterns, and pulsed and continuous wave Doppler interrogation should be performed at relevant areas of interest. The use of colour M-mode studies, in our experience, has proved to be particularly valuable in young children with rapid heart rates, since it allows a more precise temporal resolution of abnormal flow patterns. A synopsis of the standard transoesophageal views which are used in the assessment of congenital cardiac malformations is listed in Table 2.

The potential advantages and disadvantages of imaging congenital heart lesions from the oesophagus

Atrial situs and juxtaposed atrial appendages

The oesophagus has many theoretical advantages over the praecordium as a site from which to image congenital heart lesions. If a logical (i.e. sequential) approach to the diagnosis of congenital heart lesions is to be adopted then the assessment of atrial situs, the venous connections (both systemic and pulmonary) and the detailed morphology of the atrial chambers should form the first step. All these structures tend to be very poorly visualised from the praecordium. The oesophageal probe, lying in contiguity with the posterior wall of the left atrium and imaging the heart directly through the atrial blood pool, is in an excellent position to image the morphology and sites of drainage both of the pulmonary veins and the superior and inferior vena cavae. In addition the morphology of the atrial appendages (and hence atrial situs), can consistently be defined as can the complex atrial morphology associated with left or right juxta-position of the atrial appendages [3, 4].

Defects in the atrial septum

The inter-atrial septum is another structure which is best scanned from the oesophagus. Each of the four types of atrial septal defects, the secundum, primum, sinus venosus and coronary sinus defect are well defined by the oesophageal approach. *Sinus venosus atrial septal defects* are consistently defined using transverse plane transoesophageal imaging. The morphological features which characterise these defects; the superior defect in the atrial septum (roofed in part by free atrial wall), the superior vena cava over-riding the defect and the various anomalies of drainage of the right upper pulmonary vein to the superior vena cava are all well demonstrated. In our experience, imaging in the transverse plane provides the optimal approach when attempting to identify such defects; the addition of longitudinal imaging (by using a biplane probe) adds little further information. It is conceivable however that longitudinal plane imaging could be of benefit in defing complexities of drainage of the right pulmonary veins and in addition, could help to differentiate between the abnormal drainage of a right upper pulmonary vein to the superior vena cava and the drainage of a low placed hemiazygos vein to the cava, both of which can have the same appearance on transverse plane imaging.

Defects around the oval foramen (secundum atrial septal defects) are optimally studied using biplane transoesophageal imaging. It is no overstatement to say

Table 2. Summary of the sequence of imaging planes used during transoesophageal echocardiographic investigations in the assessment of congenital heart disease.

Standard examination planes	Visualisation of cardiac structures	Examples of pathology visualised
Transgastric planes	Ventricular morphology	ventricular dominance
	Ventricular relations	supero/inferior ventricles,
	Ventricular function	
	Chordal apparatus MV	parachute MV
	Inferior caval vein	interruption
	Hepatic veins	individual drainage
	Atrioventricular valves	common valve orifice
Lower oesophagus	Coronary sinus	unroofed CS
		dilated CS
	Muscular inlet septum	muscular inlet VSD
	Tricuspid valve	Ebstein's malformation
		tricuspid atresia
	4-chamber view	offsetting atrioventricular valves
		atrioventricular septal defects
		perimembranous VSD
Left atrial views	Mitral valve	valvar regurgitation
		endocarditis
	Atrial septum	patent oval foramen
		deficiencies of the oval fossa
	Pulmonary veins	anomalous connection
	Atrial chambers	atrial arrangement
		Mustard baffles
		cor triatriatum
	LV outflow tract	discrete fibromuscular obstruction
		arterial override
Mid oesophagus	Atrial septum	sinus venosus defect
		juxtaposition
	VA junction	transposition/malposition
	Superior caval vein	anomalous drainage
	Aortic valve	valvar aortic stenosis
	RV outflow tract	infundibular stenosis
	Pulmonary trunk	patent ductus arteriosus
		supravalvar stenosis
	Pulmonary arteries	palliative shunts
		·peripheral stenosis
Thoracic aorta	Aortic arch	coarctation
	descending aorta	collaterals

Legend: CS = coronary sinus; LV = left ventricle; MV = mitral valve; RV = right ventricle; RUPulmonary vein = right upper pulmonary vein; VA = ventriculo-arterial; VSD = ventricular septal defect.

Note: In the sequential analysis of congenital heart disease atrial morphology has to be determined first, thereafter atrioventricular and ventriculoarterial connections should be defined and systemic and pulmonary venous drainage determined. Only thereafter the examination should focus on the relevant lesions.

that transoesophageal imaging has provided important new insights into our appreciation of atrial septal structure and function and to defects within it. The normal transoesophageal appearance of the atrial septum when scanned in the transverse plane is of a structure which is relatively thick both superiorly and inferiorly and which is thin and multi-layered in its central portion (around the flap valve over the oval fossa). Probe-patency of the oval fossa can normally be predicted by the observation of flow information on colour flow mapping within the layers of the flap valve. This may be of clinical importance when planning subsequent catheter studies. Physiological patency of the flap valve can be tested by transoesophageal monitoring of atrial contrast flow following a peripheral venous echo-contrast injection. Both right to left shunting (the appearance of contrast bubbles in the left atrium) and left to right shunting (a negative contrast jet appearing in the right atrium from the centre of the atrial septum) can be detected. Colour M-mode studies of the flow characteristics over the oval fossa can further elucidate the complexities of physiologic inter-atrial flows. Not all of the atrial septum can be scanned using the single plane probe. The antero-inferior portion is only profiled by longitudinal scanning.

Secundum atrial septal defects are normally well visualised by transverse plane scanning [5]. In our experience, it is rare not to visualise a naturally occuring secundum defect when scanning only in the transverse plane but in 4/63 cases including 2 where there was a trivial residual inter-atrial shunt following atrial septal puncture for a mitral valvuloplasty, a defect, sited in the low antero-inferior portion of the atrial septum, was only imaged on longitudinal scanning. Transoesophageal imaging in the transverse plane determines the dimensions of the major axis (antero-posterior) of the defect while scanning in the longitudinal plane will derive the dimensions of the minor (supero-inferior) axis (Figures 1A & 1B). The assessment of these parameters is of great importance when evaluating the suitability of a secundum defect for trans-catheter closure by an occlusive device [6]. A complete biplane trans-oesophageal study should also be undertaken in such patients to determine the structures which form the defect margins and the relationship of the defect edges to the coronary sinus, the atrioventricular valves and the sites of systemic and pulmonary venous drainage. Such a detailed study should yield the information which will allow the operator to determine if a defect is suitable for transcatheter closure. The subsequent placement of all atrial (and ventricular) septal defect occlusive devices requires real-time monitoring by biplane trans-oesophageal imaging.

Other central atrial septal abnormalities better defined by transoesophageal imaging include atrial septal aneurysms (Figures 2A, 2B & 2C) and multiple fenestrations of the septum. Coronary sinus atrial septal defects are rate lesions poorly defined by either praecordial ultrasound or by angiography. Trans-oesophageal imaging appears to be the best technique to make the diagnosis. There is virtually always an associated persistent left superior vena cava

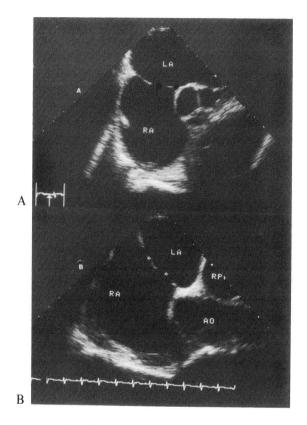

Figure 1. A: A transoesophageal transverse plane image of the atrial septum. A central defect measuring 1.2 cm is well visualised. The presence of a second defect lying immediately posterior to the aortic root was suspected but not confirmed. B: The longitudinal plane scan from the above patient clearly confirmed the presence of two discrete secundum atrial septal defects (arrowed). The inferior defect (the upper defect in this image orientation) is the defect which was poorly seen on the transverse scan.

draining to the coronary sinus with the defect in the atrial septum lying immediately adjacent to the enlarged coronary sinus orifice. In our experience the atrial component of an atrioventricular septal defect (the defect in the primun atrial septum) is equally well defined on both praecordial and transoesophageal imaging (Figure 3) [5].

Abnormalities of systemic and pulmonary venous drainage
Using a combination of transverse and longitudinal axis scanning the morphology of the systemic venous connections to the heart can be defined in every patient. The hepatic veins can be scanned from a low oesophageal or transgastric transducer position to determine if they form a confluence or whether individual hepatic veins drain separately to the atrial chambers. This latter scan is especially important in patients with atrial isomerism. A careful

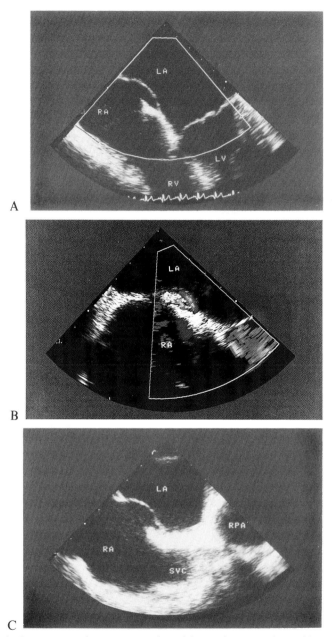

Figure 2. A: A transverse plane transoesophageal image from a patient with an atrial septal aneurysm. The aneurysmal flap valve of the oval foramen is seen to bulge into the left atrium during a valsalva manoeuvre. B: The transverse plane colour flow map from the above patient. Turbulent flow is seen to enter between the layers of the oval foramen but no shunting could be demonstrated between the atria either on colour M-mode studies or using right heart contrast echocardiography. C: A longitudinal plane image from the same patient demonstrating the aneurysmal nature of the flap valve of the oval foramen.

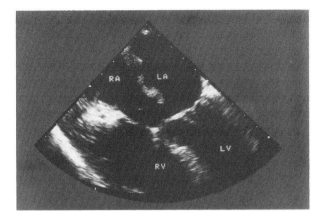

Figure 3. A transverse plane transoesophageal image from a patient with a partial atrioventricular septal defect. The primum atrial septal defect is well seen as is the posterior bridging leaflets of the common atrioventricular valve. One advantage of transoesophageal scanning in this morphology is a better definition of the subvalve chordal arrangement and insertion.

transverse axis scan of the lateral border of the left atrium should also be made to exclude a left superior vena cava. This characteristic appearance with the venous structure lying between the left atrial appendage orifice and the orifice of the left upper pulmonary vein is normally easily appreciated and the vessel can be traced to its site of drainage to the heart (normally to the coronary sinus). Longitudinal axis scanning is of additional benefit in confirming the presence of a left-sided venous structure descending with the mediastinum. Pulsed doppler sampling will confirm the venous nature of the flow and its direction.

In adult patients with normal sized atrial chambers all four pulmonary veins can be identified in approximately 96% of patients using biplane transoesophageal echocardiography. This degree of diagnostic accuracy is impossible from the praecordium. Where there is atrial dilation, the success rate with which all four veins may be visualised may be reduced but even then the two upper pulmonary veins can normally be visualised and their velocity profiles sampled using pulsed doppler. Isolated anomalies of pulmonary venous drainage, presenting in the adult age group are relatively rare and to date there have been no reports of the use of transoesophageal echocardiography in their evaluation. However, the relative additional benefits of praecordial vs. transoesophageal imaging of both cor triatriatum and isolated supramitral membrane, both presenting de novo with clinical evidence of pulmonary venous obstruction in adult patients have been described.

Transoesophageal evaluation of atrial baffle procedures
Adult patients with either a Senning or a Mustard procedure can be difficult to assess either clinically or by using praecordial echocardiography. Until the introduction of transoesophageal imaging cardiac catheterisation has remained the gold standard among investigational techniques. Transoesophageal imaging

has now changed this. A single (i.e. transverse) plane imaging study of an atrial baffle, by using a combination of 2-D imaging, colour flow mapping and selective pulsed doppler studies, can reliably identify of exclude superior limb obstruction, obstruction within the mid-portion of the systemic venous atrium, the site or sites of baffle leakage and obstruction to the drainage of individual pulmonary veins and/or obstruction within the pulmonary venous atrium itself [8]. A longitudinal axis study may contribute little to the analysis of atrial baffle function. The images obtained using this plane are often very complex (Figures 4A & 4B).

The only area within the systemic or pulmonary venous atria which is not well imaged using the transverse imaging plane is the inferior limb of the systematic venous atrium. This can be better visualised using the longitudinal imaging plane of a biplane probe.

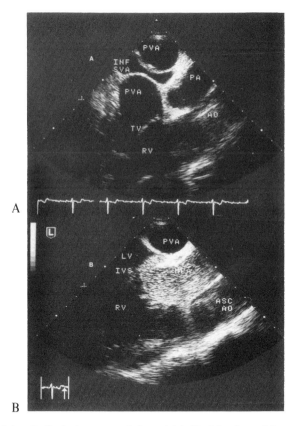

Figure 4. A: A longitudinal plane scan of the atrial baffle following a Mustard procedure. The longitudinal plane is complex to understand and all information on either superior limb obstruction, mid-baffle obstruction or baffle leakage is better obtained using transverse plane imaging. B: A peripheral venous contrast injection in the above patient. The contrast is restricted to the superior limb of the systemic venous atrium (SVA) and the inflow of the left ventricle and the main pulmonary artery. This study effectively excludes any right to left shunt at baffle level.

In view of the high incidence of clinically undetected abnormalities of baffle function which may persist or may develop late in such patients, it is our policy to routinely submit all our adult patients who have previously undergone atrial baffle procedures to a check transoesophageal study in the late post-operative period. Transoesophageal imaging can also be used in this patient group to monitor, in realtime, atrial baffle balloon dilatation procedures.

Transoesophageal evaluation of Fontan-type procedures
The spectrum of complex cardiac lesions to which a Fontan-type procedure is now applied has become very broad. The morphology of the various ways in which the surgeon re-routes the venous return is routed to the lungs is also extremely variable. The assessment of the function of the Fontan-type circulation provide perhaps the greatest diagnostic challenge to the clinician. As with atrial baffle procedures, cardiac catheterisation procedures have previously been looked on as the gold standard for the investigation of such patients. However, with the introduction of imaging from the oesophagus with its proximity to 1) the sites of systemic venous return; 2) the atria; and 3) the main and right pulmonary artery, all of which structures are involved in the construction of a Fontan connection, it seemed likely that important new information might be obtained from studying such circulations from this approach. To this end, we studied a group of children and adults who were either undergoing or who had a Fontan-type circulation [9] and compared the information derived from transverse-plane transoesophageal imaging with that obtained from either praecordial imaging or cardiac catheterisation. This study demonstrated the wealth of new and unique information which can be obtained from a transoesophageal study in such a patient group. Advantages over both praecordial imaging and cadiac catheterisation studies included: 1) improved direct visualisation of atrio-pulmonary and cavo-pulmonary connections (Figures 5A & 5B) allied to pulsed doppler evaluation of the velocity profiles throughout the connections; 2) consistent direct visualisation of both right and left-sided Glenn anastomoses and pulsed doppler interrogation of their velocity profiles; 3) a more precise evaluation (or exclusion) of any residual atrial shunting; 4) the identification or exclusion of obstruction to pulmonary blood flow; 5) the identification of pre-thrombotic flow with or without concommitant thrombus formation within the Fontan connection and the subsequent monitoring of the effects of thrombolytic therapy; 6) the direct assessment of both left atrioventricular valve and left ventricular function; 7) pulsed doppler assessment of pulmonary arterial flow patterns in the varying forms of connection with concommitant sampling of ipsilateral pulmonary vein flow patterns. The only problem areas lay in the visualisation of anterior Fontan connections using the single transverse plane transoesophageal technique and in visualising the left pulmonary artery. Both these problem areas should be circumvented by the use of the longitudinal scanning plane. Thus it is our belief that transoesophageal imaging is the diagnostic technique of first choice for use in the detailed follow-up of patients who have a Fontan connection.

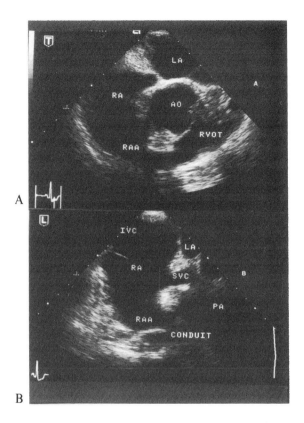

Figure 5. A: A transverse plane image of an anterior Fontan connection between the right atrial appendage (RAA) and the right ventricular outflow tract (RVOT). This connection was unusually well seen using transverse plane imaging. B: The longitudinal plane image from the above patient. Again, the connection between the RAA and the right ventricular outflow tract via a conduit is well visualised.

Transoesophageal assessment of the atrioventricular junction

While transoesophageal imaging has many advantages because of its proximity in defining posterior cardiac structures, its advantages over praecordial imaging become less clear as structures become distanced from the oesophageal probe. The current generation of probes, either single or biplane, image using crystals whose frequency is centred around 5 MHz. This allows reasonable imaging information to be acquired at depths up to 10 or 12 cm but colour flow information is much more limited at these distances. The atrioventricular junction marks the watershed for colour information from the oesophagus while adequate imaging information can usually be obtained down to the base of the papillary muscles. In terms of imaging atrioventricular function structures, transoesophageal imaging can, in our experience, better define or distinguish between: 1) absent atrioventricular connection versus an imperforate atrioventricular valve membrane; 2) the morphology of Ebsteins anomaly (both prior to or during operative repair) (Figures 6A & 6B); 3) the complex valve leaflet morphology of an atrioventricular defect; 4) a congenital cleft in the mitral valve; and, perhaps most importantly of all, can 5) identify or exclude chordal straddling in even the most complex lesions [10]. Further discussion of the complexities of the information which can be obtained on lesions of the atrioventricular junction from the oesophagus and the relative contributions of the transverse and longitudinal scanning planes is outwith the scope of this article.

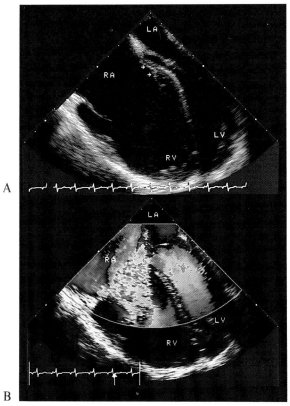

Figure 6. A: A transverse plane image from a patient with a severe form of Ebstein's malformation of the tricuspid valve. Although transoesophageal imaging can identify this anomaly, the degree of anterior leaflet displacement into the right ventricle is usually far better defined by praecordial imaging. B: A colour flow map from the above patient demonstrating severe tricuspid regurgitation whose origin is deep within the right ventricular cavity indicating the degree of valve displacement.

Transoesophageal assessment of the ventricular septum

It is relatively rare in modern cardiology practice to diagnose a congenital ventricular septal defect for the first time in the adult outpatient clinic. Where such a defect is suspected, the first line of investigation must remain a praecordial ultrasound study. With the integrated use of 2-D imaging, colour flow mapping and continuous wave doppler the morphology of an isolated restrictive defect can be determined and the associated haemodynamics defined. Transoesophageal imaging has virtually no role to play in such cases. Similarly, large non-restrictive septal defects are normally easily visualised, even in adults in whom there is a very restricted praecordial window. A combination of pulsed doppler and colour M-mode studies can help confirm the complexity of the flow patterns across such large defects. Again, in such cases transoesophageal imaging has little or no additional benefit. Indeed, single plane transoesophageal imaging is limited in its ability to assess defects in the ventricular septum in both children and adults (Figures 7A & 7B). Transverse plane imaging may not adequately profile the membranous septum and as a result false positive areas of echo drop-out may occur as the membranous

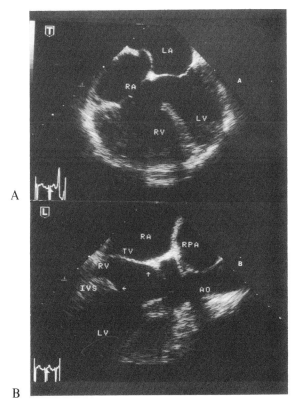

Figure 7. A: A transverse plane image of a large perimembranous confluent ventricular septal defect. Such large defects are normally well seen on transverse plane transoesophageal imaging. B: The longitudinal plane image from the above patient. Again, the anterior portion of the ventricular septal defect is well seen. Longitudinal plane imaging is of value in identifying ventricular septal defects which involve the outlet muscular septum. The longitudinal plane is also of value in defining arterial override above a ventricular septal defect.

septum moves in and out of the imaging plane. The cardiac apex, the anterior trabecular septum and the small outlet septum are other areas which are poorly visualised from the oesophagus and defects in these areas may be missed. In our experience, transoesophageal imaging can be of benefit in defining additional or multiple trabecular defects, even when these lie towards the ventricular apex. The transoesophageal approach may also be limited in its ability to identify a residual area of patch leakage following surgical closure (Table 2). This is mainly related to the material the surgeon uses for defect closure. Prosthetic material will act as a barrier to ultrasound, casting a large ultrasound shadow behind it, and thus little colour flow information will be obtained on any abnormal flow disturbance within the right ventricular cavity when imaging from the oesophagus. In this situation, large residual left to right shunts may go undetected. Even when biological material is used for the septal defect patch problems may still arise in detecting a residual shunt at ventricular

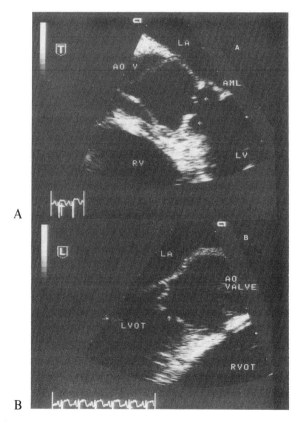

Figure 8. A: A transverse plane image from a patient with a discrete fibromuscular subaortic shelf (arrowed). B: The corresponding longitudinal plane image from the above patient. This confirms the nature of the lesion and rules out that the obstruction below the valve is due to accessory mitral valve chordae.

level. This occurs most commonly in adult patients in whom the right ventricle lies in the far field when imaged from the oesophagus and thus at, or beyond, the limits of acquisition of colour flow information.

Transoesophageal echo evaluation of the left ventricular outflow tract

Discrete fibromuscular subaortic obstruction (Figures 8A & 8B) may be a difficult entity to either identify or exclude during a praecordial ultrasound study in an adolescent or adult patient. Where any diagnostic doubt exists then a transoesophageal study is indicated. The left ventricular outflow tract is well aligned to the oesophageal ultrasound beam and all the structures which form its margins can be easily interrogated. In a prospective multi-centre study into the potential role of transoesophageal imaging in defining discrete fibromuscular sub aortic obstruction in the adolescent and adult

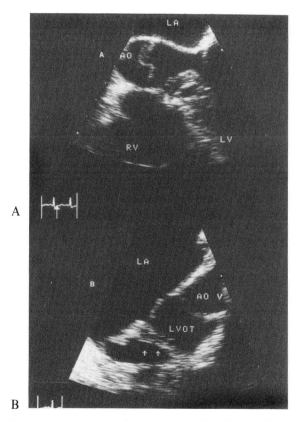

Figure 9. A: A transverse plane image from a patient with subaortic obstruction. The transverse plane study suggested that this was due to discrete fibromuscular obstruction. The longitudinal plane study gave the correct diagnosis. B: The corresponding longitudinal plane image from the above patient. This demonstrated that the subaortic obstruction was caused by accessory chordae from the mitral valve (arrowed) crossing the left ventricular outflow tract and implanting into the ventricular septum. This could not be defined by transverse plane imaging.

population, 41 patients with such a lesion were studied. This study demonstrated the superiority of the oesophageal approach in identifying the site and morphology of these often complex structures. Whereas these lesions tend to be single diaphragm-like structures in children, the findings of this study would suggest that in a proportion of patients they proliferate and become more complex with time and by adult age may develop multiple sites of insertion. In addition, the range of associated haemodynamic abnormalities (aortic regurgitation, mitral regurgitation, co-existing dynamic left ventricular outflow tract obstruction etc.) was much better defined using a combination of transoesophageal colour flow mapping and pulsed Doppler (Figures 9A & 9B, Figures 10A & 10B, Figure 11).

Transoesophageal evaluation of the semilunar valves
Although both semilunar valves can be visualised from the oesophagus the views of these structures obtained by using transverse plane imaging are

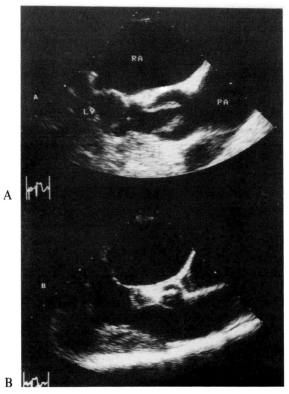

Figure 10. A: A longitudinal plane image from a patient with atrioventricular and ventriculo arterial discordance. The longitudinal plane image demonstrates a clinically unsuspected discrete fibromuscular obstruction in the left ventricular outflow tract (arrowed) and a severely stenotic bicuspid pulmonary valve. B: By probe rotation on the left, the right ventricle, right ventricular outflow tract and ascending aorta are brought into view. There is no subaortic obstruction.

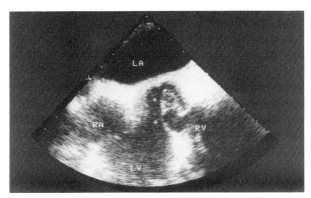

Figure 11. A transverse plane image from a patient with atrioventricular and ventriculo arterial discordance in whom a true aneurysm (arrowed) of the membranous ventricular septum was causing severe subpulmonary obstruction. This lesion was only identified during the transoesophageal study and had been missed on both praecordial imaging and angiography.

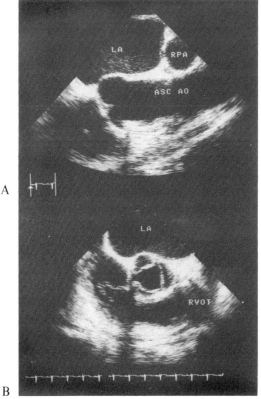

Figure 12. A: A normal longitudinal plane long axis image of the aortic valve, aortic root and ascending aorta. By fully rotating the lateral steering mechanism in the opposite direction, the image seen in Figure 12B is obtained. B: A normal longitudinal plane short axis image of the aortic valve (see above). This imaging plane will allow an excellent evaluation of aortic valve morphology and aortic valve orifice area (in non-calcific valves). See Figure 13B.

limited. Despite this, it is entirely possible to identify a bicuspid aortic valve or to identify cusp prolapse as the mechanism for valve regurgitation. The pulmonary valve is less well seen than the aortic valve and in our experience little information of value will be obtained from an imaging study restricted to the transverse plane. Biplane imaging (with the incorporation of the possibility of integrated continuous wave doppler interrogation) allows a better evaluation of both semilunar valves as the valves can be imaged in a greater number of planes (Figures 12A & 12B, Figures 13A & 13B). In addition, it would appear that the longitudinal plane allows a better alignment of the continuous wave beam to trans-oartic flow. The longitudinal plane also allows excellent visualisation of the right ventricular outflow tract as sectioned in its long axis. However, it is only possible to visualise morphology using this plane as the image of the right ventricular outflow tract always lies in the far field in adolescent and adult patients and thus beyond the depth of colour flow interrogation. Even where the great vessels are malposed or are in very

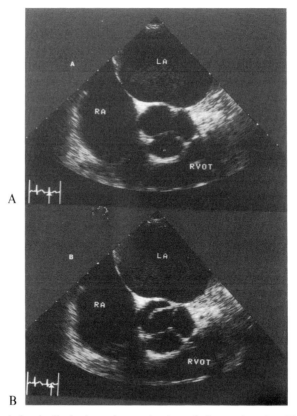

Figure 13. A: A longitudinal plane short axis view of the aortic valve. The valve appears morphologically tricuspid. However, it was functionally bicuspid (see Figure 13B). B: A late systolic frame from the above study. The apparently tricuspid valve is seen to open in a bicuspid manner with fusion of one of the valve commissures.

abnormal positions, it is our experience that biplane transoesophageal imaging can consistently determine semilunar valve morphology.

Transoesophageal evaluation of the great vessels

Of all the cardiac structures, it is in the evaluation of intra thoracic great vessel morphology that transoesophageal imaging is most limited. The ascending aorta can be visualised from the aortic root to its mid portion using transverse plane imaging. Longitudinal plane imaging increases the area of the upper ascending aorta which can be visualised and, indeed, in some cases the whole of the ascending aorta can be scanned using this plane (Table 3). Transoesophageal imaging of the ascending aorta is of value in monitoring ascending

Table 3. A comparison of intraoperative transesophegeal and epicardial echocardiography in the assessment of intracardiac morphology and haemodynamics during the surgical correction of congenital heart disease.

	Epicardial echocardiography		Transesophageal echocardiography	
	Morphological condition	Function	Morphological condition	Function
Systemic venous return	+ + +	+ +	+ +	+
Pulmonary venous return	+ +	+	+ + +	+ + +
Atrial septum	+ + +	+ +	+ + +	+ + +
Tricuspid valve	+ +	+ +	+	+ +
Mitral valve	+ + +	+ +	+ + +	+ + +
Ventricular septum	+ + +	+ + +	+	+[a]
Ventricular chambers	+ + +	+ +	+	+ + +
LVOT	+ + +	+ + +	+ + +	+
RVOT	+ + +	+ + +	−(+)[b]	−
Thoracic aorta	+ +	+ +	+	−
Pulmonary arteries	+ +	+ +	+[b]	+[b]

LVOT, Left ventricular outflow tract; RVOT, right ventricular outflow tract.
−, Inadequate; +, adequate; + +, good; + + +, excellent.
[a]Inadequate after prosthetic patch closure of ventricular septal defects.
[b]Largely dependent on the size of the acoustic window.

aortic dimensions and aortic wall morphology in patients with Marfans Syndrome (Figures 14A & 14B) and in defining or excluding congenital or acquired supra-aortic stenosis. The precise diagnostic role it may have in assessing ascending aortic pathology is yet to be defined and in the non acute-situation Magnetic Resonance Imaging or CT scanning may derive more information and this information is likely to be obtained in a manner which is much more acceptable to the patient. In a similar manner, biplane imaging allows a better assessment of the aortic arch and descending thoracic aorta. However, it has been our experience that the morphology of an aortic coarctation can be surprisingly difficult to define using the bi-plane approach. These lesions lie at the junction of the arch and descending aorta and tend to be cut obliquely by the transoesophageal ultrasound beam

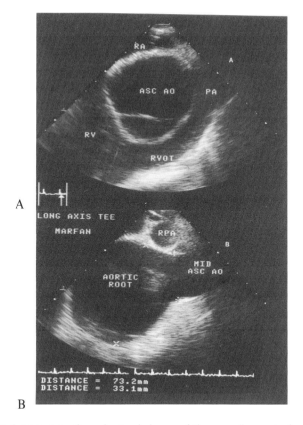

Figure 14. A: A transverse plane short axis image of the ascending aorta from a young adult with Marfan's syndrome who presented with acute chest pain. An intimal dissection flap is well visualised. B: The longitudinal plane study from the above patient clearly demonstrates the acute anterior dilatation of the aortic root and proximal ascending aorta. Cardiac surgery was performed immediately after the transoesophageal study with no other investigations being required.

using either plane. This means that the imaging appearance cannot be used to judge the severity of any narrowing which is visualised. In addition, many of these lesions are complex three dimensional structures and cannot be scanned properly from the oesophagus. Again other non-invasive imaging modalities (MRI, CT scanning) may give superior information in a more acceptable manner to the patient. Despite the problems alluded to in defining coarctation morphology, transoesophageal monitoring of balloon dilatation of a recurrent coarctation following surgery may prove to be a worthwhile procedure. Such monitoring should allow the real-time assessment of vessel wall changes and the development of complications (i.e. the occurrence of dissection etc.) during successive balloon inflations.

Transverse plane imaging can visualise the main pulmonary artery in virtually every patient. The vessel is sectioned in an oblique cut. Dilatation of the vessel can be assessed as can main pulmonary artery hypoplasia. The intrapericardial portion of the right main pulmonary artery is also easily visualised as it runs posterior to the aorta and above the superior wall of the right atrium. Central stenoses within this portion of the vessel can be visualised as can the continuous flow disturbance within the vessel associated with proximal right aorto-pulmonary shunts. The distal right pulmonary artery can be visualised in a few patients. The intrapericardial portion of the left main pulmonary artery is infrequently visualised using the transverse imaging plane as the vessel is directed almost directly posteriorly out of the scan plane. Longitudinal plane imaging is thus aligned to the vessel and will normally allow excellent images of this portion of the vessel to be obtained. Again, both morphologic and flow abnormalities within this portion of the vessel can be obtained. Again, both morphologic and flow abnormalities within this portion of the vessel can be evaluated [11, 12].

Our current evaluation of the relative advantages and disadvantages of longitudinal plane imaging versus transverse plane imaging in congenital heart disease is given in Table 4.

Table 4. Biplane tee. Advantages of longitudinal vs. transverse plane in the assessment of congenital heart disease.

Structure	New information
(a) Vena cavae	(i) Left SVC[a]
(b) Atria	(i) Pulmonary venous connections[a]
	(ii) Secundum atrial septal defects[a] (including Device closure)
	(iii) Anterior Fontan connections[a]
	(iv) Anterior conduits[a]
(c) Atrioventricular valves	(i) A-V valve morphology[a]
	(ii) A-V valve regurgitation[a]
	(iii) Chordal insertion[a]
(d) Ventricles	(i) Muscular outlet septum
(e) Outflow tracts	(i) RVOT[a]
	(ii) LVOT[a]
(f) Semilunar valves	(i) Aortic valve[a]
	(ii) Pulmonary valve
(g) Great vessels	(i) Ascending aorta (Marfan)
	(ii) A-P window
	(iii) Distal main LPA[a]
	(iv) PDA

[a]Important new information.

References

1. Sreeram N, Colli AM, Monro JL, et al. The changing role of non-invasive investigation in the preoperative assessment of congenital heart disease: A nine year experience. Br Heart J 1990;63:345–9.
2. Sreeram N, Sutherland GR, Geuskens R, et al. The role of transoesophageal echocardiography in adolescents and adults with congenital heart disease. Eur Heart J 1990;12:231–40.
3. Stümper O, Sreeram N, Elzenga NJ, Sutherland GR. The diagnosis of atrial situs by transoesophageal echocardiography. J Am Coll Cardiol 1990;16:442–6.
4. Stümper O, Rijlaarsdam M, Vargas-Barron J, Romero A, Hess J, Sutherland GR. The assessment of juxtaposed atrial appendages by transoesophageal echocardiography. Int J Cardiol 1990;29:365–71.
5. Tucillo B, Stümper O, Hess J, et al. Transesophageal echocardiographic evaluation of atrial morphology in children with congenital heart disease (accepted for publication in the Eur Heart J).
6. Hellenbrand WE, Fahey JT, McGowan FX, Weltin GG, Kleinman CS. Transesophageal echocardiographic guidance of transcatheter closure of atrial septal defect. Am J Cardiol 1990;66:207–13.
7. Stümper O, Vargas-Barron J, Rijlaarsdam M, et al. The assessment of anomalous systemic and pulmonary venous connections by pediatric transesophageal echocardiography (accepted for publication in the Br Heart J).
8. Kaulitz R, Stümper O, Geuskens R, et al. The comparative values of the precordial and transoesophageal approaches in the ultrasound evaluation of atrial baffle function following an atrial correction procedure. J Am Coll Cardiol 1990;16:686–94.
9. Stümper O, Sutherland GR, Geuskens R, Roelandt JRTC, Bos E, Hess J. Transesophageal echocardiography in the evaluation and management of the Fontan circulation. J Am Coll Cardiol 1991;17:1152–61.
10. Sreeram N, Stümper O, Kaulitz R, et al. The comparative value of surface and transesophageal ultrasound in the assessment of congenital abnormalities of the atrioventricular junction. J AM Coll Cardiol 1990;16:1205–14.
11. Omoto R, Kyo S, Matsumura M, et al. Biplane color transesophageal Doppler echocardiography (color TEE): Its advantages and limitations. Int J Card Imaging 1989;4:57–8.
12. Stümper O, Fraser AG, Ho SY, et al. Transoesophageal echocardiography in the longitudinal axis: Correlation between anatomy and images and its clinical implications. Br Heart J 1990; 64:282–8.

5. Magnetic resonance imaging

EDWARD J. BAKER

Introduction

Magnetic resonance imaging is a cross-sectional imaging technique that produces excellent images of the heart and great vessels. Interpretation of these images is made using many of the same principles used for cross sectional echocardiography. Therefore with minimal adaptation the echocardiographer can readily interpret magnetic resonance images. Understanding the technology that generates the images is generally unnecessary. An extensive understanding of normal and abnormal cardiac anatomy is essential, both when performing a magnetic resonance scan of the heart and when interpreting it. Optimum imaging of the heart can only be performed if an operator with a understanding of normal and abnormal cardiac morphology is present when the images are acquired. The correct imaging planes need to be selected with care, so that structures and features of clinical importance are imaged successfully. If the choice of imaging planes is inappropriate the study will not yield the clinical information required. It is in the study of congenital heart disease, more than anywhere else, there is no place for the use of an identical standard imaging protocol in all patients.

This applies even to the most straightforward abnormalities. Just as with cineangiography and echocardiography, the cardiologist who closely supervises the imaging procedure will achieve the best results. If he leaves the imaging to others he may well find the images of little help.

Types of magnetic resonance imaging available to the cardiologist

Most magnetic resonance images are not 'real time' they are acquired over many heart beats using electrocardiogram gating. The computer uses the electrocardiogram signal to ensure that each image is made up of data from a

John Hess and George R. Sutherland (eds.), Congenital Heart Disease in Adolescents and Adults, 79–89.
© 1992 *Kluwer Academic Publishers. Printed in the Netherlands.*

specific time in the cardiac cycle. In this way cardiac motion is not apparent in the final image. Each image is of the heart at a specific point in the cardiac cycle. Generally, for morphological imaging the stage in the cardiac cycle an image is acquired is not important. However, in functional imaging, for instance when measuring ventricular volumes, the time of the slice relative to the R wave of the electrocadiogram is critical. It can be specified by the operator.

An advantage of such magnetic resonance imaging is the good intrinsic contrast between vascular cavities and the heart or great vessels. In addition, magnetic resonance images can be acquired in any plane. Early studies of magnetic resonance imaging in congenital heart disease were limited to standard transverse, sagittal or coronal phases [1–5]. The newer generation of high field strength magnetic resonance imaging systems can exploit the ability to image in oblique planes. Some of the planes used will be immediately recognisable to the echocardiographer, but with magnetic resonance imaging there are no limitations on the imaging planes that can be used. Careful use of imaging planes most appropriate to both the anatomy of the malformed heart and to the clinical problem has realised the full potential of magnetic resonance imaging [6–9]. Again, it must be emphasised that failure to show important aspects of the anatomy is most frequently due to the choice of inappropriate imaging planes, rather than to any intrinsic weakness in the imaging technique.

The most frequently used cardiac images are termed 'spin echo' images. These are high resolution, static images. The cardiac structures appear light and the vascular cavities dark. These images are the most important for the study of cardiac anatomy because of this excellent intrinsic contrast and because of their high resolution.

Moving, but not real time, images can be acquired by setting up cine loops of a series of spin echo images acquired at different times during the cardiac cycle. To do this with spin-echo images involves a very long acquisition time and so is not clinically practical. The term cine magnetic resonance imaging usually refers to 'fast field echo' images which are lower resolution and have less intrinsic contrast than spin echo images. The advantage of these images is that a cine loop of fast field echo images can be acquired with an acceptable imaging time. The fast field echo imaging sequence generates an increased signal intensity from flowing blood. Moving blood, therefore, appears light and the contrast with the vascular structures is poor. However, turbulent blood flow appears dark. A cine loop of such images has been described as 'pseudo-angiographic' because of the superficial similarity to a cine angiogram. This is a false analogy. It is important to realise that the images are cross-sectional and are therefore fundamentally different from cine angiograms. This type of cine magnetic resonance imaging has been used to calculate ventricular volumes and ejection fractions, demonstrate the presence of high velocity flow through the sites of aortic coarctation and identify the presence of tricuspid, mitral and aortic regurgitation [10, 11].

Echoplanar imaging is a real time magnetic resonance imaging technique. Fast imaging acquisition times are used so that cardiac images can be acquired without the need for electrocardiogram gating. Development of the echoplanar technique is likely to be important in the future, but as yet, the resolution has not approached that obtained with spin echo imaging [12, 13].

Three dimensional reconstruction is already being used in examination of the central nervous system and has recently been used in patients with congenital heart disease [14]. The method of image reconstruction requires a series of up to 20 images to be acquired in a transverse plane encompassing structures between the base of the heart and the aortic arch. The scanning times range from 59 to 120 min. Processing these images currently takes 4 to 6 h. The final images are surface and endocast volume three dimensional reconstructions of the heart and great vessels that can be viewed in any plane or orientation. If imaging and processing times can be reduced three dimensional reconstruction may supersede current cross-sectional imaging formats. For the time being, however, it is not a practical clinical tool.

Imaging of specific cardiac abnormalities

In the few years that magnetic resonance imaging has been available much experience has now been gained in the imaging of different aspects of cardiac morphology and many cardiac malformations. The majority of cardiac malformations can be imaged satisfactorily and magnetic resonance imaging is undoubtedly a versatile and widely applicable technology.

Atrial arrangement, venous connections

Magnetic resonance imaging is able to display all the structures relevant to the identification of situs [9]. For instance, polysplenia or asplenia and the relationship between the abdominal aorta and the inferior caval vein to each other and the spine can be identified in transverse images through the upper abdomen. Interruption of the hepatic section of the inferior vena cava with azygous or hemiazygous continuation has been identified as well as direct communication between the hepatic vein and the right atrium. Bronchial morphology can be displayed in coronal images of the thorax. It is also possible to image the atrial appendages. The right atrial appendage is often demonstrated in transverse planes. The left atrial appendage is demonstrated in oblique or coronal sagittal imaging planes. Images of the appendages are usually associated with areas of increased signal intensity, most probably due to their high fat content. Magnetic resonance imaging is an excellent technique for imaging abnormal venous connections, whether they coexist with atrial isomerism [15] or not. Systemic venous connections are very well shown. Pulmonary venous connections can also be successfully imaged, although more skill is needed. The reason for this is that respiratory motion prevents adequate imaging of the distal pulmonary veins. Only the insertion of the veins into atria or other structure is demonstrated. Where all the pulmonary veins do no drain to the same site great care needs to be taken to ensure that all are imaged. This being said, magnetic resonance imaging by a skilful operator is probably the best way of demonstrating abnormal pulmonary venous drainage currently available.

Atrial septum and interatrial communications

The atrial septum can be imaged in a number of planes (Figure 1). Interatrial defects including secundum defects, sinus venous defects and atrioventricular septal defects can be demonstrated [16, 17]. However, failure, to image the floor of a thin oval fossa can lead to a false diagnosis of an atrial septal defect. This is a problem comparable to that of 'drop out' with echocardiography. Care must be taken to image the atrial septum in a plane truly orthogonal to the oval fossa, to avoid this mistake. Oblique cuts through the atrial septum are most likely to lead to the false identification of an atrial septal defect. As a general rule structures, such as this, which can be distorted by oblique imaging should be demonstrated in at least two orthogonal planes.

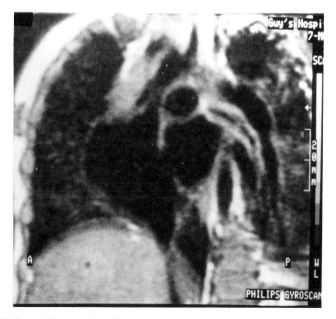

Figure 1. This is an oblique sagittal slice through the heart to show the atrial septum in short axis. Anteriorly, to the left, is the right atrium, the entry of the superior vena cava and inferior vena cava is clearly seen. There is a clear secundum atrial septal defect in the septum in the centre of the image. Posterior to this is a smaller left atrium, above which the right pulmonary artery is seen in short axis.

Atrioventricular connections and atrioventricular valves

Magnetic resonance imaging can readily identify concordant, discordant, double inlet left and right ventricle and absent right and left atrioventricular connections [6]. In addition, the mode of atrioventricular connection can usually be identified in those patients in whom atrial and ventricular morphology has previously been established. Straddling, common, imperforate and overriding atrioventricular valves can also be imaged (Figure 2). Imaging of atrioventricular valves may be improved by adjusting the timing of the imaging within the cardiac cycle. This is well worth trying if initial imaging is unsatisfactory. However, spin echo images are static and do not demonstrate valve function. Cine fast field echo images can demonstrate valve motion and incompetence. In practice, echocardiography is usually superior for the study of atrioventricular valve function.

Ventricular morphology

Magnetic resonance imaging can clearly differentiate the morphologically smooth walled left ventricle from the morphologically trabeculated right ventricle. This is usually achieved in images taken in a transverse plane [6]. It is also possible to quantify relative ventricular proportions, if necessary ventricular volumes can be measured. In addition, magnetic resonance provides a new insight in the imaging of ventricular septal defects (Figure 2). Imaging planes can be obtained parallel to the inlet and trabecular ventricular septum. These images effectively give a face on view of the greater part of the septum which can precisely localise defects and can identify multiple defects [7].

Ventriculo-arterial connections

Magnetic resonance imaging can be used to establish the mode of ventriculo-arterial connection. In an extensive series we have been able to correctly identify a wide variety of connections including concordant, discordant, double outlet right ventricle, common arterial trunk and single arterial connections [18]. Magnetic resonance imaging has proved to be of particular benefit in patients with double outlet of one ventricle. Not only is the relationship of the great arteries defined, but the relationship of the arterial valves to ventricular septal defects can be determined with a new degree of precision.

The great arteries

Magnetic resonance imaging now has a well established role in the study of the aortic arch and the pulmonary arteries. There is no doubt that it is in this area that magnetic resonance imaging has proved to be of the most benefit.

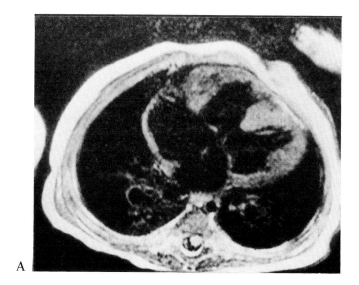

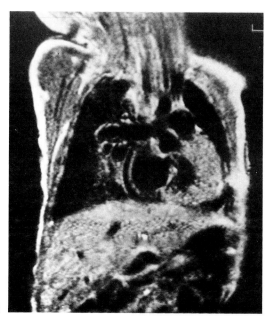

Figure 2. A: transverse four chamber slice through a heart with an atrioventricular septal defect. There is also a secundum atrial septal defect. The morphology of the anterior (top) right ventricle and the posterior left ventricle are well seen. There are large atrial and ventricular components to the defect. The common valve is clearly seen bridging the defect. B: An oblique coronal slice in a heart with an atrioventricular septal defect. This shows the ventricular septum face on. The large ventricular defect can be clearly seen, bordered superiorly by the superior and inferior bridging leaflets of the common valve. The right pulmonary artery is particularly well seen in this image.

Oblique sagittal images in the plane of the aortic arch can show the anatomy of the whole arch in one image, although in some patients, particularly adults, several neighbouring slices are needed to show the whole arch (Figure 3). Great care is required if the arch is tortuous not to misinterpret the images. When there appears to be an obstruction, it is essential to image the suspect area in at least two orthogonal planes to avoid this. Coronal planes through the area of interest are usually best for this, but standard transverse planes can also be of value.

The pulmonary trunk and the branch pulmonary arteries are usually first seen in transverse slices through the upper mediastinum (Figure 4). Just as with the aorta it is essential to obtain additional views. An oblique sagittal view is planned through the left pulmonary artery and an oblique coronal view through the right pulmonary artery. In this way excellent views of the pulmonary arteries can be obtained. Just as with the pulmonary veins, the pulmonary arteries cannot be seen once they have entered the lungs, because of respiratory motion. However, it is possible to image both arteries up to their first bifurcation, and in the case of the left pulmonary artery, often well beyond.

In patients with major aorto-pulmonary collateral arteries, these are seen at their origin from the aorta, but their course and distribution cannot be determined since they are so tortuous. This is perhaps one area where selective angiography will continue to be necessary [19].

Conclusions

Magnetic resonance imaging can be used to study all aspects of cardiac morphology, in the majority of areas it can provide morphological detail as good, if not better, than other non-invasive and invasive imaging techniques. It is to be expected that with more widespread availability and improved imaging software magnetic resonance imaging will become the definitive technique for study the morphology of the heart in life.

Clinical role of magnetic resonance imaging

While magnetic resonance can image most congenital cardiac defects, it will not replace echocardiography as the first line non-invasive imaging technique. For older patients with poor echocardiographic windows it is likely to have an increasingly important role. This is particularly true for those with suspected abnormalities of the great arteries and venous connections. But, undoubtedly magnetic resonace imaging is of value in the study of intracardiac defects and particularly so where the relationships between structures are complex. The question 'When do you use magnetic resonance imaging?' is therefore easy to answer. It should be considered in all cases where echocardiographic studies fail to provide an adequate morphological diagnosis. Appropriate use of magnetic resonance imaging should significantly reduce the need for

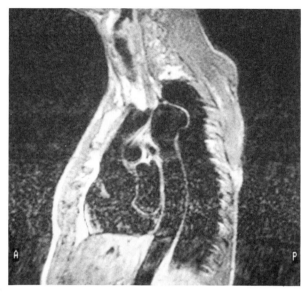

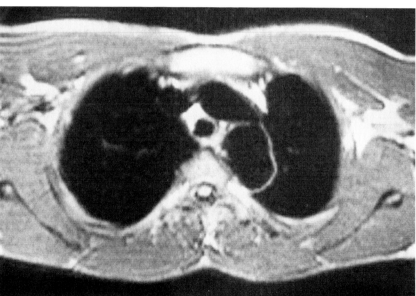

Figure 3. A: An oblique sagittal image in an adult with a coarctation repaired with a Dacron patch. The anatomy of the arch is clearly seen. There is a large aneurysm at the site of the patch. There is a suggestion of obstruction proximal to this. B: A transverse image through the area that appeared obstructed in Figure 3A. There clearly is an obstruction in the transverse arch, proximal to the patch repair.

cineangiography. Indeed, the cardiologist who has access to both echocardiography and magnetic resonance imaging should only rarely require cineangiography for the diagnosis of congenital heart disease.

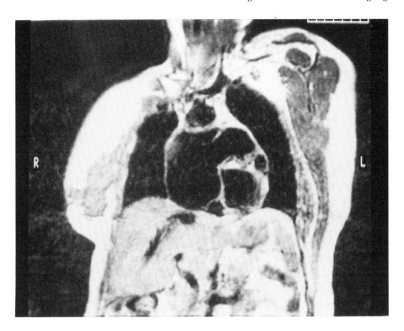

A

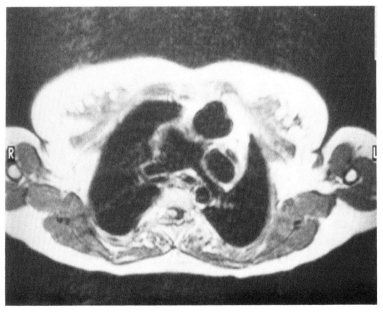

B

Figure 4. A: A coronal image through the right atrium in a patient following a Fontan operation for tricuspid atresia. The cavity of the dilated atrium occupies much of the heart in this slice. The right atrial appendage forms the conduit to the pulmonary arteries. The left atrial appendage can just be seen beneath the tip of the right appendage. B: A transverse slice through the right atrial appendage in the same patient as Figure 4A. The anastomosis to the pulmonary arteries is seen as are the two pulmonary arteries themselves. The ascending aorta is anterior and to the left of the pulmonary trunk.

Problems

Since it is an electrocardiogram gated technique, an irregular heart beat can seriously degrade the images. Metal implants, including sternal wires and vascular clips can produce substantial artefacts. Magnetic resonance imaging is possible with most prosthetic valves, since few modern valves contain ferromagnetic materials. Electronic pacemakers are a contraindication to imaging. A minority of patients find the imaging procedure frightening and need reassurance, occasionally sedation. There is, however, no discomfort for the patient and they can be accompanied by the a parent or friend. Magnetic resonance imaging carries no risk and does not use ionising radiation. It is, therefore, ideally suited to patients with congenital heart defects who may require many imaging studies over a period of years.

References

1. Higgins CG, Byrd BF, Farmer DW, Osaki L, Silverman NH, Cheitlin MD. Magnetic resonance imaging in patients with congenital heart disease. Circulation 1984;70:851-60.
2. Fletcher BD, Jacobstein MD, Nelson AD, Riemenschneider TA, Alfidi RJ. Gated magnetic resonance imaging of congenital cardiac malformations. Radiology 1984;150:137-40.
3. Jacobstein MD, Fletcher BD, Nelson A, Goldstein S, Alfidi J, Riemenschneider TA. ECG-gated nuclear magnetic resonance imaging: Appearance of the congenitally malformed heart. Am Heart J 1984;107:1014-20.
4. Higgins CB, Stark D, McNamara MT. Magnetic resonance imaging of the heart: A review of the experience in 172 subjects. Radiology 1985;155:671-9.
5. Didier D, Higgins CB, Fischer MR, Osaki L, Silverman NH, Cheitlin MD. Congenital heart disease: gated magnetic resonance imaging in 72 patients. Radiology 1986;158:227-35.
6. Smith MA, Baker EJ, Ayton V, Parsons JM, Ladusans EJ, Maisey MN. Magnetic resonance imaging of the infant heart at 1.5 T. Br J Radiol 1989;62:367-70.
7. Baker EJ, Ayton V, Smith MA, et al. High field strength magnetic resonance imaging of ventricular septal defects in infants. Br Heart J 1989;62:305-10.
8. Baker EJ, Ayton V, Smith MA, et al. High field strength magnetic resonance imaging of coarctation of the aorta in infants. Br Heart J 1989;62:97-101.
9. Parsons JM, Baker EJ. The use of magnetic resonance imaging in the investigation of infants and children with congenital heart disease: Current status and future prospects. Int J Cardiol 1990;29:263-75.
10. Chung KJ, Simpson IA, Glass R, Sahn DJ, Hesselink JR. Cine magnetic resonance imaging after surgical repair in patients with transposition of the great arteries. Circulation 1988;77:104-9.
11. Simpson IA, Chung KJ, Glass RF, Sahn DJ, Sherman FS, Hesselink J. Cine magnetic resonance imaging for evaluation of anatomy and flow relations in infants and children with coarctation of the aorta. Circulation 1988;78:142-8.
12. Chripsin A, Small P, Rutter N, et al. Transectional echoplanar imaging of the heart in cyanotic congenital heart disease. Pediatr Radiol 1986;16:293-7.
13. Chrispin A, Small P, Rutter N, et al. Echoplanar imaging of normal and abormal connections of the heart and great vessels. Pediatr Radiol 1986;16:289-92.
14. Laschinger JC, Vannier MW, Gutierrez F, et al. Preoperative three dimensional reconstruction of the heart and great vessels in patients with congenital heart disease. J Thorac Cardiovasc Surg 1988;96:464-73.

15. Fisher magnetic resonance, Hricak H, Higgins CB. Magnetic resonance imaging of developmental venous anomalies. Am J Roentgenol 1985;145(4):705–9.
16. Lowell DG, Turner DA, Smith SM, et al. The detection of atrial and ventricular septal defects with electrocardiographically synchronized magnetic resonance imaging. Circulation 1986;73:89–94.
17. Jacobstein MD, Fletcher BD, Goldstein S, Riemender TA. Evaluation of atrioventricular oseptal defect by magnetic resonance imaging. Am J Cardiol 1985;55:1158–61.
18. Parsons JM, Baker EJ, Hayes A, et al. Magnetic resonance imaging of the great arteries in infants. Int J Cardiol 1990;28:73–85.
19. Rees SO, Somerville J, Underwood SR. Magnetic resonance imaging of the pulmonary arteries and their systemic connections in pulmonary atresia; comparison with angiographic and surgical findings. Br Heart J 1987;58:621–6.

6. Interventional cardiac catheterization for primary or residual congenital cardiac lesions

MAARTEN WITSENBURG

Introduction

Interventional catheterization techniques, especially balloon valvuloplasty and angioplasty have gained increasing popularity during the recent years as an alternative for surgical intervention for a variety of primary or residual lesions in congenital cardiac disease. After the initial report by Kan e.a. in 1982 of successful balloon dilatation of pulmonary valve stenosis, application of the technique for a wide range of congenital cardiac malformations has been reported [1–7]. The indications included primary congenital malformations as well as residual lesions after surgery. Valvular pulmonary stenosis, valvular aortic stenosis, aortic coarctation and recoarctation are the most frequently reported diagnoses. In these the place of the technique in relation to surgery becomes clear, although longer term follow up reports are limited. In most reports the age range is wide, from infancy to adulthood.

Next to balloons for dilatation procedures, new devices have become available for occlusion of primary or residual congenital lesions. Transcatheter closure of the ductus arteriosus is now feasible in many patients [8, 9]. Small series have been reported on the use of occluding devices for atrial and ventricular septal defects [10–12].

Balloon valvuloplasty and angioplasty

Technical considerations

Interventional catheterization in children and adolescents is preferably performed under general anaesthesia. Shortly before and during the actual intervention the FiO_2 is raised to warrant adequate oxygen reserve. For valvuloplasty and aortic angioplasty initially heparin 100 IU/kg i.v. is administered

91

John Hess and George R. Sutherland (eds.), Congenital Heart Disease in Adolescents and Adults, 91–102.
© *1992 Kluwer Academic Publishers. Printed in the Netherlands.*

to prevent clotting and to diminish local problems at the entry site of the catheter. Heparin administration can be repeated at a lower dose if the procedure takes long. A transfemoral venous or arterial approach is mostly used. After haemodynamic evaluation of the lesion biplane angiography is performed. Exact measurements of the stenotic site or valve annulus is essential for proper selection of the balloon size. A guide wire is placed through the site of the lesion with the tip of the wire generously behind the stenosis. For the type of lesions to be dilated mostly balloons are used with diameters between 6 and 25 mm, usually mounted on catheters with French sizes 5–8. The considerable size of the deflated balloon cathethers precluded the use of sheaths in most of the paediatric and adolescent patients. More recently low profile balloon catheters with diameters up to 14 mm have been manufactured, fitting sheaths with French size 7.5. If the catheter size precludes the use of a sheath, the vessel entry should be gently dilated before the balloon catheter is introduced. The size of the balloon chosen depends on the type and size of malformation. After proper positioning of the balloon over a wire guide 0.035″ or 0.038″, the dilatation is performed under direct fluoroscopy (Figure 1). Inflation time is kept relatively short, in valvular lesions up to 10 seconds, in angioplasty slightly longer.

The moment the waist disappears deflation should be performed as soon as possible to restore cardiac output. After removal of the balloon catheter the result of the intervention is evaluated by repeat haemodynamic and angiographic studies. Bleeding from the groin after removal of the catheters is controlled by attentive local manual compression. Especially after a trans-

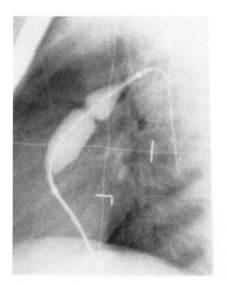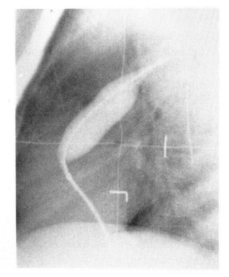

Figure 1. Balloon valvuloplasty for valvular pulmonary stenosis. During inflation the waist disappears.

arterial procedure close observation of the patient with respect to femoral artery complications such as bleeding or thrombosis is necessary [13, 14].

Valvular pulmonary stenosis

Balloon valvuloplasty for isolated valvular pulmonary stenosis has proven to be successful, and is now regarded by many as the primary choice of treatment. Several reports have shown good relief of the pressure gradient, including a recent report by the VACA-registry (Valvuloplasty and Angioplasty of Congenital Anomalies) of more than 750 procedures, which also highlights the wide acceptance of the technique as an alternative for surgical valvulotomy [2].

The indication for treatment is a continuous wave Doppler derived gradient of 50 mmHg or more. In our experience the invasively measured gradient in these patients undergoing general anaesthesia may at times be less than 40 mmHg. In these cases confirmation of the severity of the stenosis may be obtained by measurement of the valve area.

The relief of the gradient is obtained by commissural splitting [15]. In general the gradient diminishes by at least 60%. In patients with dysplastic pulmonary valves, as frequently observed in Noonan's syndrome, the result may be less satisfying. The right ventricular hypertrophy and high contractile state of the ventricle may result in a substantial residual infundibular stenosis which disappears with time (Figure 2) [16]. There is generally no need for beta-blocking agents.

With the use of balloons with a diameter 1.2–1.3 times the size of the angiographically determined annular valve ring, good results are obtained without trauma to the valve annulus itself. When a large valve ring is present a

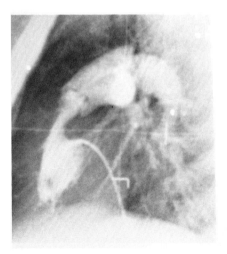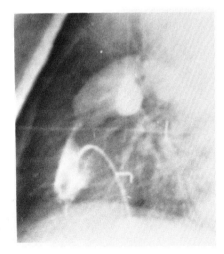

Figure 2. Severe systolic infundibular narrowing before pulmonary valvuloplasty, which increased after the dilatation. Spontaneous regression occurred within months.

double balloon technique may be used. Dilatation will frequently result in some regurgitation of the pulmonary valve, but the low pressure in the pulmonary artery system precludes the haemodynamic significance of this. Improper balloon positioning may result in injury of the tricuspid valve. Transoesophageal echocardiography as a guide for catheter positioning may be helpful in preventing this complication [17].

The successful reduction in valve gradient is maintained at longer term follow up [18].

Valvuloplasty for valvular pulmonary stenosis is effective and after infancy the complication rate is low. Restenosis is infrequent and mostly amenable for repeat dilatation [19]. Also in adult patients this technique has proven to be safe and effective. Now the treatment for valvular pulmonary stenosis is so easy, a trend is observed towards accepting also mild stenosis as an indication for treatment. Mild valvular pulmonary stenosis can be progressive in a subgroup of paediatric patients, however in adults it is not a progressive disease. Therefore, justification of treatment in this group is still questionable.

Valvular aortic stenosis

The success of pulmonary valvuloplasty prompted several groups to use this technique for treatment of aortic valve stenosis as well. However, there is still considerable debate over the value of this treatment as an alternative for surgery (3, 20, 21]. The main concern is the risk of a considerable increase in valve regurgitation.

At present we consider the presence of ST-T segment changes at rest or during bicycle ergometry and/or a continuous wave Doppler gradient of 60 mmHg or more as an indication for treatment. Syncope is seen as an indication for treatment, even if the other criteria are not met.

Technically the procedure is not as simple as in pulmonary valvuloplasty. Passing the wire guide through the small valve opening may be time consuming. The use of a coronary artery catheter is frequently helpful in passing the valve. A more than grade 2 angiographic aortic regurgitation is generally regarded as a contraindication for treatment, because of the risk of an increase in valve regurgitation. The baloon diameter should be 0.9–1.0 times the valve annulus, to minimize this risk. Stabilizing the balloon during dilatation can be difficult, however part of this problem can be overcome by the use of longer balloons and the use of stiffer wire guides. Several reports, including the VACA-registry, show a 60 percent reduction in gradient. The mean reduction in Doppler gradient after valvuloplasty in our own experience is 50 percent, which reduction persists at a mean follow up of 2.8 years (Figure 3) [22]. Half of our patients underwent a surgical valvulotomy earlier on. The gradient reduction in this group did not differ from the patients in whom valvuloplasty was the first intervention. The major complication is valvular regurgitation. In our experience the incidence of substantial valve regurgitation after valvulo-plasty is 20 percent and some increase in regurgitation may be observed during

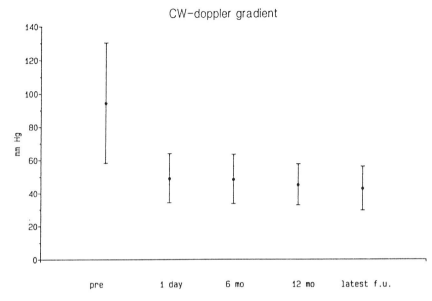

Figure 3. Continuous wave Doppler determined transvalvular gradient in 21 patients (age 1 month to 15.9 years) before(pre) aortic valvuloplasty and at 1 day, 6 months, 12 months and at latest follow-up [22] (reprinted with permission from the publisher).

follow up (Figure 4). Regurgitation necessitated valve replacement in three patients within two years after the valvuloplasty. All three patients had undergone earlier surgical valvulotomy. Femoral artery thrombosis is a complication seen especially in younger children which can be handled with streptokinase or surgery with reasonable success [13]. The introduction of balloon catheters with a low profile, especially if used with a sheath, will likely diminish the incidence of this complication.

One of the main reasons to perform balloon valvuloplasty for valvular aortic stenosis is postponing surgical intervention in the growing individual. This is a less strong argument in the adolescent patient. If valvulotomy would be the surgical alternative, dilatation could be of value. But only valve replacement, preferably a homograft or a pulmonary autograft, will completely relief the obstruction and will give the better outlook for preservation of left ventricular function. Once the third or fourth decade is reached, calcification of the congenital abnormal valve will play a major role in causing the obstruction. In the calcified aortic valve the effect of valvuloplasty is very limited and not long lasting.

Aortic coarctation and recoarctation

Since the publication of the initial experience by Lock in 1983, many reports on balloon angioplasty for aortic coarctation and recoarctation have been published [4, 5, 23–25]. The effect is obtained by tearing the intima and part of

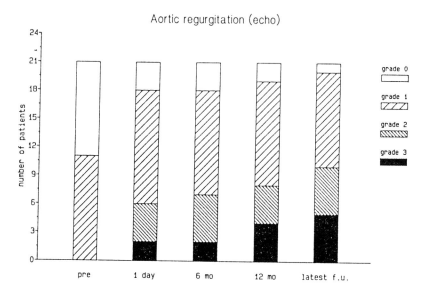

Figure 4. Aortic valve regurgitation determined with echo-doppler in 21 patients before(pre) valvuloplasty and at 1 day, 6 months, 12 months and at latest follow-up [22] (reprinted with permission from the publishers).

the media, which has led to concern in relation to pseudo-aneurysm formation, especially in those patients that did not underwent prior surgery [26].

Diminished femoral artery pulses and a substantial pressure difference between the upper and lower part of the body, eventually combined with upper body hypertension are the indications for treatment of a native or a residual coarctation.

Angioplasty results in a mean reduction of the pressure gradient of 75 percent and generally the coarctation diameter doubles. The results in coarctation and recoarctation are comparable in this respect. A residual gradient over 20 mmHg is observed in 10–20 percent of the patients. Restenosis may occur and is especially observed after dilatation of native coarctation. Fatal complications are rare. Recently a fatal rupture of the aorta in an attempt to dilate a recoarctation after a patch angioplasty has been reported [27]. Due to the transarterial approach, femoral artery thrombosis and bleeding are known complications, especially in younger children. Aneurysm formation is likely to be a more important problem in patients who did not have prior surgery, because of the lack of circumferential scar tissue that may prevent its occurrence. Because aneurysm formation can occur with time, imaging of the dilated segment during follow up after the angioplasty is necessary, either with biplane angiography, or with magnetic resonance imaging. In our own experience we observed one small aneurysm in 30 patients who underwent angioplasty for recoarctation, with no progression at follow up at one and two years. However, the long term consequences of aneurysm formation are not known yet. If surgery is available for unoperated (native) coarctation, it is doubtful whether angiopasty is really an alternative for this indication. In our experience balloon angioplasty for aortic recoarctation is a valuable alternative for surgical reintervention.

Other malformations

Balloon angioplasty has been used for many other lesions with variable success [7]. These include conduit obstruction, pulmonary branch stenosis, systemic-pulmonary shunts, systemic venous obstructions, subvalvular aortic stenosis etc. Some of these emerge as a reasonable indication from the series that have been reported.

Baffle obstruction after Mustard or Senning-repair for transposition

A atrial switch operation for transposition of the great arteries, either Mustard or Senning, may be complicated by an obstruction of the venous pathways due to narrowing of the intra-atrial baffle. This will result in either systemic or pulmonary venous congestion. Angioplasty for systemic venous obstruction is successful in the majority of patients (Figure 5) [7]. However, the number of procedures published is very limited. The indication for treatment is not well described. In our own experience, in many patients after a Mustard repair a mean pressure difference of 2 mmHg between the systemic veins and the

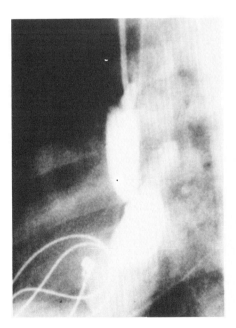 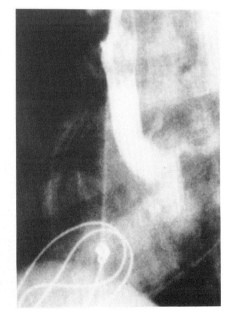

Figure 5. Severe narrowing of the superior baffle in a patient after Mustard repair of transposition of the great arteries, with successful result of the dilatation.

systemic venous atrium is a regular finding. In the 7 patients in whom balloon angioplasty was performed the mean venous pressure gradient decreased from 8 to 3 mmHg. In one patient complete obstruction of the superior baffle prevented dilatation. We did not observe any complications but a non fatal cardiac tamponade has been observed once (Dr. M. Talsma, personal communication).

Periferal pulmonary stenosis

The VACA-registry reported a large series of angioplasty for branch pulmonary artery stenosis [6]. Primary stenoses as well as branch stenoses after earlier surgery have been dilated. Balloon angioplasty results only in a moderate reduction in pressure difference and some increase in vessel diameter. Local complications such as vessel perforation and rupture have been observed. Death has been reported in 3% of the patients. However, one should realize that some of the more distal stenoses are not amenable for surgery.

Recently the use of redilatable intravascular stents is suggested for pulmonary artery branch stenosis. This technique is currently under investigation.

Right ventricular outflow tract obstruction

Dilatation of right-sided conduit obstruction due to a stenosed prosthetic valve has been reported to be successful in 30% of the patients, postponing surgical intervention in some of them [28].

Balloon dilatation of the right ventricular outflow tract in tetralogy of Fallot has been advocated [29]. The partial relief of the outflow tract obstruction should increase the pulmonary bloodflow, resulting in an increase of oxygen saturation thereby postponing or eliminating the need for systemic-pulmonary artery shunting. However, it does not lead to substantial growth of the valve annulus, so a transannular patch will still be needed at the time of surgical correction [30]. Many centers however, will prefer a one-stage surgical approach in tetralogy, leaving little place for balloon valvuloplasty.

Acquired obstructions between the right ventricle and the pulmonary artery may complicate surgical repair. Hancock prostheses may obstruct due to calcification and excessive intimal proliferation. Also with the use of homografts there is a risk of obstruction, especially at the proximal or distal anastomosis. Whenever the stenosis is very localized, balloon angioplasty may be performed, but the results are frequently not satisfying at the longer term.

Dilating pulmonary artery stenosis after an arterial switch operation has been reported to be disappointing [20].

Fixed subaortic-stenosis

In this type of subvalvular aortic stenosis a spiralling fibrous shelf in the left ventricular outflow tract is causing the obstruction. Balloon dilatation may result in partial relief of the gradient but also in this lesion it is likely that surgery is the more effective way of treatment [7]. Since the shelf often is morphologically related to the mitral valve apparatus, the dilatation procedure may result in mitral valve damage and should therefore in our opinion not be performed.

Stenosed shunts

Increasing the pulmonary bloodflow by systemic-pulmonary shunting is useful for temporary or definitive palliation in a variety of congenital cardiac malformations. In most institutions a modified Blalock-Taussig anastomosis is the preferable procedure. During growth a stenosis may occur on either the proximal or distal site. These stenoses may be dilated successfully [32, 33].

Occluding devices

Technical considerations

Occlusion of a ductus arteriosus with the Rashkind PDA occluder is preferably performed by the transvenous route [8]. The morphology of the ductus is outlined with an aortogram with special attendance of the relation of the ductus to the anterior tracheal wall. A large sheath is positioned through the ductus into the aorta. The double umbrella device is delivered by means of a special delivery system (Figure 6). After angiographic control of its position the device is relieved.

   As a variant on the double umbrella principle, a clamshell device is manufactured for the closure of atrial defects. This device is currently under clinical investigation [11]. There is a major role for transoesophageal echocardiography in monitoring guidance of the placement of this device [34].

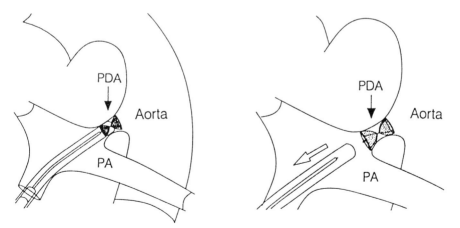

Figure 6. Positioning and relief of a occluding device for a patient ductus arteriosus (PDA = patent ductus arteriosus; PA = pulmonary artery).

Patent ductus arteriosus

The use of an occluder as alternative for surgical closure of a patent ductus arteriosus has been applied in several institutions. There is general agreement that a ductus arteriosus should be closed not only because of the left-to-right shunt but especially because of the associated risks for endocarditis. There is a considerable morphological variation of the ductus which may interfere with the success of the procedure [35]. In our own experience this technique is effective in the majority of the patients. Dislodgement of the device seldomly occurs after positioning. Due to the fact that the complete closure of the ductus may take some time, a residual shunt is frequently found at echochardiograhic examination early after the intervention. This may lead to heamolysis in a rare case [36]. Most of these residual leaks will have closed spontaneously within three months. Endocarditis prohylaxis is maintained for at least three months after the intervention, and until Doppler-echocardio-graphic examination has revealed complete closure and normal flow patterns in the pulmonary artery and descending aorta [37].

Atrial and ventricular septal defects

The experience of umbrella closure of atrial septal defects is limited. It has been applied as well for secundum type atrial septal defects as for residual atrial shunts after earlier surgery [11]. The device can only be used in centrally positioned atrial septal defects with a limited diameter. For secundum type atrial septal defects this means that half of the patients would eventually benefit from such an approach. At present the use of an umbrella device for the closure of a ventricular septal defect is investigational. One study reported the use of an occluding device in muscular ventricular septal defects which were difficult to handle surgically [12]. The technique is less standard than in a ductus or atrial septal defect, and more studies will be needed before the role of umbrella closure for ventricular septal defects is known.

Conclusion

Although the follow up of balloon valvuloplasty and angioplasty for congenital lesions is limited, it is likely to be the definitive treatment for valvular pulmonary stenosis and at least a substantial part of the patients with aortic recoarctation. In valvular aortic stenosis it postpones valve replacement in the majority of patients but the increase of valvular regurgitation remains of concern. In unoperated coarctation and tetralogy we prefer surgery as the initial approach. In the majority of the other indications balloon angioplasty may be valuable in postponing surgical intervention.

Umbrella closure of the ductus arteriosus is becoming a standard approach in several institutions. The results sofar are promising but the follow up is limited. The use of an occluder for atrial and ventricular septal defects needs further investigation.

References

1. Kan JS, White jr. Rl, Mitchell SE, et al. Percutaneous balloon valvuloplasty: A new method for treating congenital pulmonary valve stenosis. N Engl J Med 1982; 302:540–2.
2. Stanger P, Cassidy SC, Girod DA, Kan JS, Lababidi Z, Shapiro SR. Balloon pulmonary valvuloplasty: Results of the valvuloplasty and angioplasty of congenital anomalies registry. Am J Cardiol 1990;65:775–83.
3. Rocchini AP, Beekman RH, Shachar GB, Benson L, Schwartz D, Kan JS. Baloon aortic valvulopasty: Results of the valvulopasty and angioplasty of congenita aomalies registry. Am J Cardiol 1990;65:784–9.
4. Tynan M, Finley JP, Fontes V, Hess J, Kan J. Balloon angioplasty for the treatment of native coarctation: results of the valvuloplasty and angioplasty of congenital anomalies registry. Am J Cardiol 1990;65:790–2.
5. Hellenbrand WE, Allen HD, Golinko RJ, Hagler DJ, Lutin W, Kan J. Balloon angioplasty for aortic recoarctation: Results of the valvuloplasty and angioplasty of congenital anomalies registry. Am J Cardiol 1990;65:790–2.
6. Kan JS, Marvin WJ, Bass JL, Muster AJ, Murphy J. Balloon angioplasty-branch pulmonary artery stenosis: Results of the valvuloplasty and angioplasty of congenital anomalies registry. Am J Cardiol 1990;65:798–801.
7. Mullins CE, Latson LA, Neches WH, Colvin EV, Kan J. Balloon dilation of miscellaneous lesions: results of valvuloplasty and angioplasty of congenital anomalies registry. Am J Cardiol 1990;65:802–3.
8. Rashkind WJ, Mullins CE, Hellenbrand WE, Tait MA. Nonsurgical closure of patent ductus arteriosus: clinical application of the Rashkind PDA Occluder System. Circulation 1987;75:583–92.
9. Ali Kkan MA, Mullins CE, Nihill RH, et al. Percutaneous catheter closure of the ductus arteriosus in children and young adults. Am J Cardiol 1989;64:218–21.
10. Lock JE, Cockerham JT, Keane JF, Finley JP, Wakely PE, Fellows KE. Transcatheter umbrella closure of congenital heart defects. Circulation 1987;75:593–9.
11. Rome JJ, Keane JF, Perry SB, Spevak PJ, Lock JE. Double umbrella closure of atrial defects. Initial clinical applications. Circulation 1990;82:751–8.
12. Bridges ND, Perry SB, Keane JF, et al. Preoperative transcatheter closure of congenital muscular ventricular septal defects. N Engl J Med 1991;324:1312–7.
13. Brus F, Witsenburg M, Hofhuis WJD, Hazelzet JA, Hess J. Streptokinase treatment for femoral artery thrombosis after arterial cardiac catheterisation in infants and children. Br Heart J 1990;63:291–4.
14. Burrows PE, Benson LN, Williams WG, et al. Iliofemoral arterial complications of balloon angioplasty for systemic obstructions in infants and children. Circulation 1990;82:1697–704.
15. Ettedgui JA, Ho SY, Tynan M, et al. The pathology of balloon pulmonary valvoplasty. Int J Cardiol 1987;16:285–93.
16. Fontes VF, Esteves CA, Sousa, JEMR, Silva MVD, Bemborn MCB. Regression of infundibular hypertrophy after pulmonary valvuloplasty for pulmonic stenosis. Am J Cardiol 1988;62:977–9.
17. Stümper O, Witsenburg M, Sutherland GR, Cromme-Dijkhuis A, Godman MJ, Hess J. Transoesophageal echocardiographic monitoring of interventional cardiac catheterization in children. J Am Coll Cardiol 1991;18:1506–14.
18. McCrindle BW, Kan JS. Long-term results after balloon pulmonary valvuloplasty. Circulation 1991;83:1915–22.

19. Khan MAA, Al-Yousef S, Moore JW, Sawyer W. Results of repeat percutaneous balloon valvuloplasty for pulmonary valvar restenosis. Am Heart J 1990;120:878–81.
20. Vogel M. Benson LN, Burrows P, Smallhorn JF, Freedom RM. Balloon dilatation of congenital aortic valve stenosis in infants and children: short term and intermediate results. Br Heart J 1989;62:148–53.
21. Shaddy RE, Boucek MM, Sturtevant JE, Ruttenberg HD, Orsmond GS. Gradient reduction, aortic valve regurgitation and prolapse after balloon aortic valvuloplasty in 32 consecutive patients with congenital aortic stenosis. J Am Coll Cardiol 1990;16:451–6.
22. Witsenburg M, Cromme-Dijkhuis AC, Frohn-Mulder IME, Hess J. Short and mid-term results of balloon valvuloplasty for valvular aortic stenosis in children. Am J Cardiol. 1992;69:945–50.
23. Cooper RS, Ritter SB, Rothe WB, Chen CK, Griepp R, Golinko RJ. Angioplasty for coarctation of the aorta: Long-term results. Circulation 1987;75:600–4.
24. Rao PS, Wilson AD, Chopra PS. Immediate and follow-up results of balloon angioplasty of postoperative recoarctation in infants and children. Am Heart J 1990;120:1315–20.
25. Hess J, Mooyaart El, Busch HJ, Bergstra A, Landsman MLJ. Percutaneous transluminal balloonangioplasty in restenosis of coarctation of the aorta. Br Heart J 1986;55:459–61.
26. Brandt III B, Marvin Jr. JM, Rose EF, Mahoney LT. Surgical treatment of coarctation of the aorta after balloon angioplasty. J Thorac Cardiovasc Surg 1987;94:715–9.
27. Balaji S, Oommen R, Rees PG. Fatal aortic rupture during balloon dilatation of recoarctation. Br Heart J 1991;65:100–1.
28. Waldman JD, Schoen FJ, Kirkpatrick SE, Mathewson JW, George L, Lamberti JJ. Balloon dilatation of porcine bioprosthetic valves in the pulmonary position. Circulation 1987;76:109–14.
29. Battistessa SA, Robles A, Jackson M, Miyamoto S, Arnold R, McKay R. Operative findings after percutaneous pulmonary balloon dilatation of the right ventricular outflow tract in tetralogy of Fallot. Br Heart J 1990;64:321–4.
30. Sreeram N, Saleem M, Jackson M, et al. Results of balloon pulmonary valvuloplasty as a paliative procedure in tetralogy of Fallot. J Am Coll Cardiol 1990;18:159–65.
31. Saxena A, Fong LV, Ogilvie BC, Keeton BR. Use of balloon dilatation to treat supravalvar pulmonary stenosis developing after anatomical correction for complete transposition. Br Heart J 1990;64:151–5.
32. Qureshi SA, Martin RP, Dickinson DF, Hunter S. Balloon dilatation of stenosed Blalock-Taussig shunts. Br Heart J 1989;61:432–4.
33. Rao PS, Levy JM, Chopra PS. Balloon angioplasty of stenosed Blalock-Taussig anastomosis: Role of balloon-on-a-wire in dilating occluded shunts. Am Heart J 1990;120:1173–8.
34. Hellenbrand WE, Fahey JT, McGowan MD, Weltin GG, Kleinman CS. Transesophageal echocardiographic guidance of transcatheter closure of atrial septal defect. Am J Cardiol 1990;66:207–13.
35. Krichenko A, Benson LN, Burrows P, Moes CAF, McLaughlin P, Freedom RM. Angiographic classification of the isolated, persistently patent ductus arteriosus and implications for percutaneous catheter occlusion. Am J Cardiol 1989;63:877–80.
36. Ladusans EJ, Murdoch I, Franciosi J. Severe haemolysis after percutaneous closure of a ductus arteriosus (arterial duct). Br Heart J 1989;61:548–50.
37. Ottenkamp J, Hess J, Talsma MD, Buis-Liem TN. Protrusion of the device; a complication of catheter closure of patent ductus arteriosus (accepted for publication in the Br Heart J).

7. Pulmonary atresia

NYNKE J. ELZENGA

Introduction

In cases with pulmonary atresia there is no direct outlet from the heart into the pulmonary arteries. The pulmonary blood supply is provided either by a ductus arteriosus or by aortopulmonary collateral arteries. Since there are mayor differences in both clinical presentation and management between pulmonary atresia with an intact ventricular septum and pulmonary atresia with a VSD it has become common practice to divide cases with pulmonary atresia into these two groups.

Pulmonary atresia with intact ventricular septum

In pulmonary atresia with an intact ventricular septum the atresia usually consists of an imperforate pulmonary valve, but may include the right ventricular infundibulum as well. The pulmonary trunk and the pulmonary arteries are patent in virtually all cases, and well developed in the majority. The size of the right ventricle ranges from enlarged in cases with severe tricuspid incompetence to extremely hypoplastic. Right ventricular to coronary artery communications, commonly associated with coronary artery stenoses, may be present in cases with a hypoplastic right ventricle and a competent tricuspid valve [1].

The blood supply to the pulmonary arteries is by a ductus arteriosus in all cases. Although earlier autopsy studies [2] revealed the ductus to be persistent in approximately 10% of the cases with pulmonary atresia and an intact ventricular septum, long term natural survival has not been reported. Apparently even a persistent duct will show contraction shortly after birth, leading to severe cyanosis of the neonate and prompting immediate intervention. The management consists of prostaglandin infusion to reopen the ductus, followed

John Hess and George R. Sutherland (eds.), Congenital Heart Disease in Adolescents and Adults, 103–115.
© 1992 *Kluwer Academic Publishers. Printed in the Netherlands.*

by either the institution of an aortopulmonary shunt or corrective surgery. The choice of the procedure largely depends on the size of the right ventricle [3] and the presence of associated anomalies. An eventual biventricular correction will be possible in the majority of the patients. In some others a Fontan type of repair will be a possibility.

Both early and late mortality are still high; however, an increasing number of these patients may be expected to reach adulthood [4]. The relevance of discussing this lesion in the setting of adolescent and adult congenital heart disease, is that late postoperative problems will occur in those surviving into adulthood. In the cases that underwent a biventricular repair long term prognosis will be determined by residual lesions, such as right ventricular outflow tract obstruction or significant pulmonic and tricuspid insufficiency [5], as well as by RV function. The problems associated with a long-term Fontan circulation will be discussed elsewhere (chapter 8).

Pulmonary atresia with VSD

In pulmonary atresia with a VSD, or a complex intracardiac anomaly, the atresia usually involves the subpulmonic outflowtract as well as the valve level. The pulmonary trunk and arteries are patent in the majority of the cases, but some degree of hypoplasia is the rule rather than the exception. The right and left pulmonary arteries are usually confluent, but may be non-confluent. Complete atresia of the pulmonary trunk and one or both pulmonary arteries, however, is not exceptional.

The degree of underdevelopment of the central pulmonary arteries is closely related to the alternative sources of the pulmonary blood supply. This source may be a ductus arteriosus, bilateral ducts, or major aortopulmonary collateral arteries (MAPCA's). A ductus arteriosus and MAPCA's are mutually exclusive: a lung is either supplied by a duct or by MAPCA's [6].

Pathology

Pulmonary atresia with VSD and a ductus arteriosus

Approximately half of the cases with pulmonary atresia and a VSD (in former days also called: 'Fallot with pulmonary atresia') will present with a ductus arteriosus, supplying confluent pulmonary arteries. Contrary, virtually all the cases with pulmonary atresia and VSD in combination with a complex intracardiac defect have this type of pulmonary blood supply. The latter group will not be discussed in this chapter.

Twenty-five percent of the ducts in pulmonary atresia and VSD are reported to be persistent [2]. However, as in pulmonary atresia with an intact ventricular septum, survival into adult life on a patent ductus is exceptional.

At birth, the pulmonary arteries are patent in the majority of the patients and the peripheral distribution of these pulmonary arteries is complete. This means, all lung segments are supplied by these central pulmonary arteries; there are no arborization anomalies as in the cases with pulmonary blood supply by MAPCA's. However, abnormalities of the central pulmonary arteries are common. Congenital pulmonary artery stenoses, located at the site of entry of the ductus arteriosus into the pulmonary artery are found in 60% of the cases with pulmonary atresia and a VSD and ductal pulmonary blood supply [7]. A pulmonary artery stenosis may become atretic and thus lead to acquired non-confluence of the pulmonary arteries (Figure 1).

Pulmonary atresia with VSD and MAPCA's

Aortopulmonary collateral arteries, that are present at birth and occur as an alternative route of blood supply to the peripheral pulmonary vascular bed are nowadays usually referred to as MAPCA's or Systemic Collateral Arteries. The

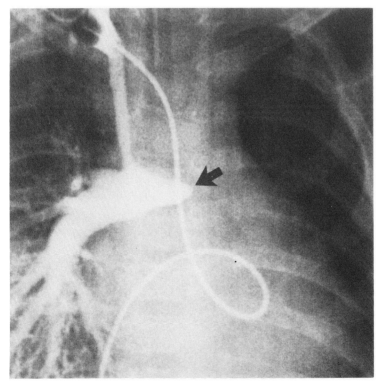

Figure 1. Contrast injection into a modified right Blalock-Taussig shunt in a patient with pulmonary atresia and a VSD. The pulmonary arteries were confluent at the time of the shunt operation, however, a localised narrowing at the origin of the left pulmonary artery (LPA) had been present. The arrow points to the site of the aquired atresia of the LPA.

former term is preferable, since the latter does not explicitly distinguish between the congenital and the acquired collaterals. Acquired collaterals develop after birth in patients with diminished pulmonary blood flow and in older patients will frequently coexist with the MAPCA's or with the ductus arteriosus. They are commonly enlarged bronchial, mediastinal or pleural arteries, that anastomose in the periphery of the lungs with the pulmonary arterioles. They are usually numerous and follow a tortuous course (Figure 2).

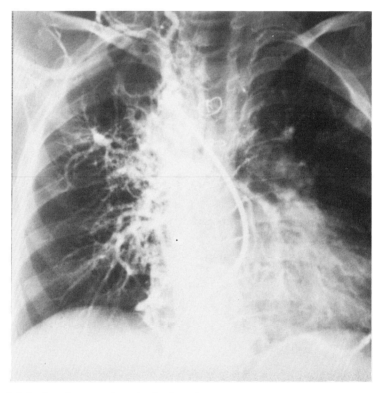

Figure 2. Injection of contrast into the distal aortic artch, showing the opacification of numerous tortuous aquired collateral arteries to the right lung. Note the patient had a previous sternotomy, which possibly stimulated the development of these collateral arteries.

MAPCA's, on the contrary, are not enlarged normal bronchial arteries, but are considered to be persistent early embryonic vessels. The former term: 'bronchial collaterals' is nowadays abandoned. However, there is still dispute about the relationship between MAPCA's and bronchial arteries. Some authors described bronchial arteries as separate vessels, unrelated to the MAPCA [8], whereas others [9] demonstrated bronchial arteries originating from a MAPCA. In a recent study of autopsy and angiographic material at the Mayo Clinic, in which the author participated, the relationship between the bronchial arteries and the MAPCA's was reevaluated. We confirmed the findings of Liao et al. [9] in demonstrating bronchial arteries originating from a MAPCA (Figure 3). However, it appeared, that certain types of MAPCA were more likely to give rise to bronchial arteries than others. Bronchial branches were particularly common in MAPCA's originating from a subclavian artery. Thus far an explanation for this association has not been given.

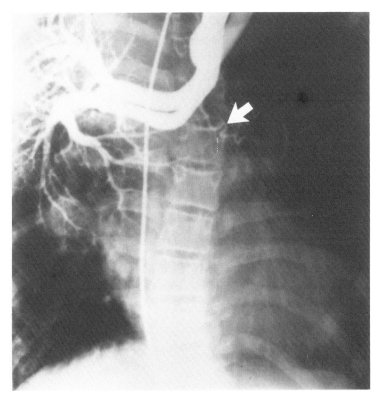

Figure 3. Major aorto-pulmonary collateral artery (MACPA) originating from the left subclavian artery. The MAPCA supplies the upper lobe of the right lung. A bronchial artery to the left lung (arrow) originates from the MAPCA.

The pulmonary vascularization patterns in patients who have MAPCA's are highly variable. The number of MAPCA's per patient, the site of origin of the MAPCA from the systemic circulation and the different modes of connexion between the MAPCA and the pulmonary vascular bed offer numerous possibilities. The resulting patterns are complex and hardly predictable in an individual patient, despite many attempts to categorize MAPCA's [9–11]. In the Mayo Clinic material mentioned above the number of MAPCA's per patient varied from 1 to 6. The majority of the MAPCA's originated from under the aortic arch or from the thoracic descending aorta (85%), 10% came from a subclavian artery and the remainder from ther sources (carotid artery, abdominal aorta, etc.). The extrapulmonary course of the MAPCA's showed marked variation. Some coursed ventrally to the bronchi, others dorsally. When crossing the midline, this might be ventral or dorsal to the esophagus, and sometimes in between the esophagus and the trachea. There was no correlation between the extrapulmonary course of the MAPCA and the type of anastomosis with the pulmonary vascular bed. Most MAPCA's anastomosed end-to-end with a lobar or segmental pulmonary artery, thus, as an end-artery, directly supplying a part of the distal pulmonary vascular bed (Figure 4). In addition some gave off one or more sidebranches, that anastomosed sideways or via a loop with a 'true' central pulmonary artery (Figure 5). The former type is called a non-communicating, the latter a communicating MAPCA. The number of communications per MAPCA [9] and the number of communicating MAPCA's per patient is highly variable. More exceptionally MAPCA's

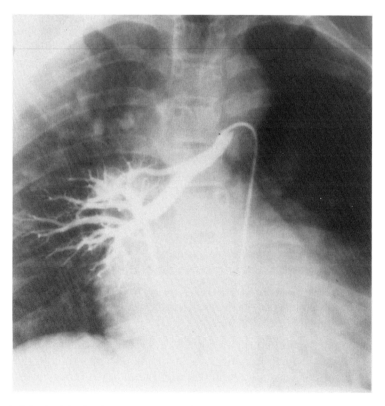

Figure 4. Selective injection into a non-communicating MAPCA, supplying the right middle lobe. The MACPA communicates with the peripheral pulmonary vascular bed in a manner comparable with that of the MAPCA in Figure 3. There is no opacification of a true central pulmonary artery.

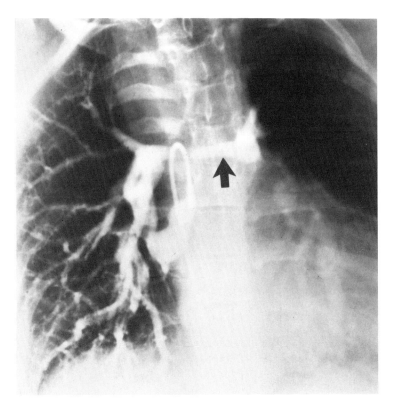

Figure 5. Selective injection into a communicating MAPCA. The central pulmonary arteries (arrow) are confluent, but hypoplastic. The arborisation of the right pulmonary artery is virtually normal, whereas the arborisation of the left pulmonary artery is incomplete.

anastomose directly in an end-to-side manner with a central pulmonary artery. These MAPCA's have no 'branches of their own', as the other types.

Central pulmonary arteries are present in $\pm\frac{3}{4}$ of the patients. These may be confluent or non-confluent. The communication of these central pulmonary areries may be with one or with several MAPCA's and the site of communication may be located at hilar, lobar or segmental level. The size of the central pulmonary arteries is thought to correlate with the amount of blood flowing through them [12].

In patients with MAPCA's and central pulmonary arteries arborization abnormalities of this central pulmonary artery system are the rule rather than the exception. Autopsy series revealed 50–75% of the bronchopulmonary segments to be connected to the central pulmonary arteries [8, 9].

Although stenoses at the origin of the MAPCA from the systemic circulation were encountered in some cases, stenosis at the site of the anastomosis of the MAPCA with the peripheral pulmonary arterial bed was the commonest finding. These latter stenoses may be located far peripherally, well within the lung itself. The histology of the MAPCA's is as variable as their course. Some are muscular arteries from their origin from the aorta till their anastomosis with the pulmonary vascular bed; others are mainly elastic or musculo-elastic. Stenoses occur in all types, a correlation between the type of vessel wall and stenoses could not be established. Stenoses are progressive with time, due to secondary intimal proliferation, and may eventually lead to complete occlusion of a MAPCA.

The peripheral pulmonary arterial bed is originally normal in distribution and histology, irrespective of its mode of supply: via the central pulmonary artery, a MAPCA or both. However, with increasing age of the patient, changes secondary to alterations in blood flow will take place. Areas supplied by stenotic MAPCA's will be underperfused and have a low pressure in the distal pulmonary arteries. In areas supplied by non-obstructed MAPCA's with severe pulmonary overflow, pulmonary vascular obstructive disease will develop.

Diagnosis

The patients with pulmonary atresia, VSD and ductal pulmonary blood supply will present as neonates with severe cyanosis, due to a constricting ductus. The clinical symptoms in patients with pulmonary blood supply by MAPCA's vary with the amount of pulmonary blood flow. Marked cyanosis will be the presenting symptom in cases with poorly developed or stenotic MAPCA's. In cases with large, unobstructed MAPCA's cyanosis will be virtually absent and heart failure may occur in infancy. However, in the majority of the patients cyanosis will become apparent with time, due to progressing stenoses or pulmonary vascular disease.

At physical examination the heart is usually hardly or only moderately enlarged. The first heart sound is normal and the second sound single. A soft ejection systolic murmur may be audible at the left sternal border, but a harsh pulmonary stenosis murmur (as in tetralogy of Fallot) is absent. Continuous murmurs, often most prominent over the back, may be present and are caused by the flow across the collaterals. However, continuous murmurs are often absent, both in patients with seriously impaired pulmonary blood flow due to stenotic MAPCA's and in those with pulmonary arterial hypertension.

The chest X-ray may reveal the classical boot shaped heart with diminished pulmonary vascular markings, or the typical irregular appearance of the pulmonary vascular markings in cases with MAPCA's [12].

Echocardiography will readily establish the VSD, the enlarged aorta overriding the defect, and the right ventricular hypertrophy. Definitive exclusion of a patent right ventricular outflow tract to the pulmonary artery may be difficult in older patients, even with Doppler colourflow mapping. When present, the central pulmonary artery can often be visualized in the neonate and infant, whereas this is often impossible in older patients. In infants other features, like the presence or absence of a ductus arteriosus under the aortic arch, are readily appreciated. However, even in infants it may be difficult to distinguish a ductus originating from a subclavian artery from a MAPCA. Colourflow mapping may be of great help in identifying several MAPCA's, originating from the descending aorta. All these echocardiographic features are difficult to establish in older children and often impossible to identify in adults.

Cardiac catheterization and selective angiography is the procedure of choice to delineate the pattern of pulmonary blood supply in cases with MAPCA's. This study should be performed in a specialized unit, by a cardiologist, aware of the complex pathology to be anticipated. Hemodynamic measurements are mainly performed to establish ventricular function and pulmonary resistance. The latter is, however, hazardous in the presence of multifocal pulmonary blood supply [13]. Angiography should identify the source of pulmonary blood supply to all the lung segments. In general, all MAPCA's have to be injected selectively to demonstrate the presence or absence of communications with a central PA. Communications can be detected by direct opacification of a pulmonary artery from the injection of contrast material into a MAPCA, or by the demonstration of 'wash-out' of contrast material by unopacified blood from another MAPCA. If selective injections fail to demonstrate a central PA system, pulmonary venous wedge angiography may be performed. Stenoses in the MAPCA's, as outlined above, should be identified and the presence or absence of bronchial artery branches established.

In older children and adults marked degrees of cyanosis and polycythemia are frequently present. It is hazardous to fast these patients for a prolonged period of time and use large amounts of contrast material, since this may lead to dehydration. Moreover, there is an increased risk of thromboembolic complications and acute renal failure in these patients. If the pulmonary vascular anatomy is complex, it may therefore be advisable to divide the study into 2 or more separate sessions. During the periods of fasting and during the catheter study a continuous intravenous fluid delivery is mandatory [12].

Natural history

When the pulmonary blood supply is by a ductus arteriosus, the patient will become severely cyanosed as a neonate, prompting immediate surgical intervention. Contrary, the natural history of pulmonary atresia with VSD and MAPCA's is variable and depends mainly on the adequacy of the pulmonary blood supply through the MAPCA's. Given the complexity of the pathology, however, the course is relatively favorable. Severe cyanosis in a neonate is uncommon. Contrary to the ductus arteriosus, with its tendency to acute closure, the MAPCA's remain patent after birth. Many patients will however become progressively cyanosed during childhood, due to failure of the MAPCA's to grow with the growth of the child and progression of the stenoses in the MAPCA's. The peripheral pulmonary vascular bed supplied by the MAPCA's may show suboptimal growth as well. Nevertheless, some patients may survive into adulthood [14].

Surgical treatment

The initial management of the neonate with ductal pulmonary blood supply will be prostaglandin infusion, followed by the surgical creation of an aortopulmonary shunt in the majority of the infants. Different types of aortopulmonary shunt operations have been used in the past. The descending aorta to left pulmonary artery anastomosis (Pott's shunt) has nowadays been abandoned, since it caused pulmonary hypertension in many cases. The ascending aorta to right pulmonary artery anastomosis (Waterston shunt) may also cause pulmonary arterial hypertension. In addition, both shunts commonly lead to kinking and stenosis of the pulmonary artery used. The Blalock-Taussig shunt, either the original right subclavian artery to right pulmonary artery end-to-side anastomosis or with interposition of some prosthetic material, is the procedure of choice nowadays in most institutions. Subsequently, corrective surgery will be performed in the majority of the cases.

Until recently, the surgical possibilities for treatment of patients with pulmonary atresia, VSD and MAPCA's were mainly dependent on the presence of the central pulmonary arteries. The usual initial surgical treatment consisted of a shuntoperation to the central pulmonary artery. The use of a right ventricular to central pulmonary artery outflow reconstruction as a palliative procedure, rather than a shuntoperation, has also been reported [15]. Patients without a central pulmonary artery were considered inoperable.

The vital importance of possible arborization anomalies of the central PA has been acknowledged. Only those patients with central pulmonary arteries of adequate size, that were free of significant proximal stenoses and that were connected to a sufficient number of bronchopulmonary segments were considered candidates for corrective surgery in one large series [16]. The group reporting on the palliative outflow reconstruction [15] stated, that the patients were considered candidates for complete repair, if adequate growth of the central pulmonary arteries occurred and the pulmonary artery distribution was to more than the equivalent of one lung. This appeared to be the case less than 50% of the cases.

Corrective surgery for pulmonary atresia and VSD has been performed with various methods to establish continuity between the right ventricle and the central pulmonary arteries: valvotomy alone, transannular patching, non valved conduits and heterograft or homograft valved conduits. The majority of the patients had undergone one or more shuntoperations prior to the correction. The results of complete repair have been encouraging, but considerably worse than those in patients with tetralogy of Fallot and a patent right ventricular outflow tract. A five year survival of 76%, 10 year of 69% and 20 year of 58% has been reported after complete repair [17]. The size of the central pulmonary arteries appears to be a mayor determinant of the risk involved in the repair. A high immediately post repair RV/LV pressure ratio is associated with a poor outcome. A recent study reemphasizes the vital importance of arborization anomalies in pulmonary atresia with VSD and

MAPCA's: late post repair pulmonary artery pressure and resistance are inversely related to the number of broncho-pulmonary segments connected to the central pulmonary artery [18].

Those patients formerly considered inoperable – the ones with very hypoplastic central pulmonary arteries and severe arborization anomalies and those without central pulmonary arteries – may nowadays also become candidates for surgery. The only possibility for an eventual repair in these patients, is when their sources of pulmonary blood supply can be 'unifocalized'. The same is true for a number of patients, who have iatrogenic non confluence of the central pulmonary arteries, due to previous palliative surgery [12]. The concept of unifocalization emerged in the late 1970s and thus far few results have been reported. One group reported 26 patients that underwent unifocalization as a first palliative procedure. Three of these patients subsequently underwent complete repair, while another 4 are considered candidates for repair. Four patients died, 13 survived, but were no candidates for repair. Only 5 of these latter 13 were clinically improved thanks to the palliative unifocalization procedure. The authors wonder whether the unifocalization is, in fact, a realistic goal.

Another group [19] reported 38 patients who underwent unifocalization procedures (26 of whom had had no previous surgery), 35 of them survived. Twenty-three of these patients underwent complete repair, 2 of which died. Another 8 patients are awaiting surgery and only 4 are no candidates for further surgery.

Management of the individual patient

Although the surgical possibilities for patients with pulmonary atresia, VSD and MAPCA's have improved considerably in recent years, the question how to manage an individual patient remains a difficult one. As outlined above, given the complexity of the lesion, the natural history of pulmonary atresia, VSD and MAPCA's is relatively favorable. The results of surgical treatment thus far, do not seem to justify an aggressive approach in all patients presenting with this defect in infancy. However, an initial non-surgical approach will transform some patients into unsuitable candidates for later repair, by allowing secondary changes of the peripheral vasculature and thrombosis of the central pulmonary arteries [11] to develop.

Todays adults with this lesion present as a heterogenous group. Some will have undergone corrective surgery, however, they will need a lifelong medical supervision. A variety of late sequelae has been reported after surgical correction of Fallot's tetralogy, including: endocarditis, rhythm disturbances, residual RV hypertension and poor RV function [20]. After correction of pulmonary atresia and VSD at least a similar number of problems has to be anticipated.

Those that have undergone palliative surgery may be inoperable as a result of iatrogenic damage to their central pulmonary arteries, such as excessive stenosis or non confluence of their central pulmonary arteries or pulmonary vascular disease. Others, however, may benefit from the present surgical possibilities, such as unifocalization procedures, and may even become candidates for complete repair. Whether the risk involved in the surgical procedure is justified in an individual patient, depends on the number and the complexity of the procedures involved and on the actual clinical condition of the patient. The same is true for those patients, that never had any previous surgical procedures. Counseling in a specialized adult congenital heart disease unit is necessary, before any decision on surgical intervention is taken. The surgery should only be performed in these specialized units, by surgeons experienced in the treatment of this specific type of complex congenital heart disease.

Acknowledgements

The author is grateful to Paul Julsrud, William Edwards and Bob Feldt of the departments of cardiac radiology, pathology and pediatric cardiology of the Mayo Clinic (Rochester, USA) for their help in the study of the cases of pulmonary atresia and VSD. The illustrations were provided by Paul Julsrud.

References

1. Gittenberger-de Groot AC, Sauer U, Bindl L, Babic R, Essed CE, Buhlmeier K. Competition of coronary arteries and ventriculo-coronary arterial communications in pulmonary atresia with intact venricular septum. Int J Cardiol 1988;18:243–58.
2. Cassels DE, Bharati S, Lev M. The natural history of the ductus arteriosus in association with other congenital heart defects. Perspect Biol Med 1975;18:541–70.
3. De Leval M, Bull C, Start J, Anderson RH, Taylor JFN, Macartney FJ. Pulmonary atresia and intact ventricular septum: Surgical management based on revised classification. Circulation 1982;66:272–80.
4. Hawkins JA, Thorne JK, Boucek MM, et al. Early and late results in pulmonary atresia and intact ventricular septum. J Thorac Cardiovasc Surg 1990;100:492–7.
5. Kaplan S, Adolph RJ, Murphy DJ. Pulmonic valve stenosis. In: Roberts WC, editor. Adult congenital heart disease. Philadelphia: FA Davis Company, 1987:477–91.
6. Thiene G, Frescura C, Bini RM, Valente C, Galluci V. Histology of pulmonary arterial supply in pulmonary atresia with ventricular septal defect. Circulation 1979;60:1066–74.
7. Elzenga NJ, v Suylen RJ, Frohn-Mulder I, Essed CE, Bos E, Quaegebeur JM. Juxtaductal pulmonary artery coarctation: An underestimated cause of branch pulmonary artery stenosis in patients with pulmonary atresia or stenosis and a ventricular septal defect. J Thorac Cardiovasc Surg 1990;100:416–24.
8. Haworth SG, Macartney FJ. Growth and development of the pulmonary circulation in pulmonary atresia with ventricular septal defect and major aortopulmonary collateral arteries. Br Heart J 1980;44:14–24.
9. Liao P, Edwards WD, Julsrud PR, Puga FJ, Danielson GK, Feldt RH. Pulmonary blood supply in patients with pulmonary atresia and ventricular septal defect. J Am Coll Cardiol 1985;6:1343–50.
10. Rabinovitch M, Herrera de Leon V, Castaneda AR, Reid L. Growth and development of the pulmonary vascular bed in patients with tetralogy of Fallot with or without pulmonary atresia. Circulation 1981;64:1234–49.

11. Shimazaki Y, Maehara T, Blackstone EH, Kirklin JW, Bargeron LM. The structure of the pulmonary circulation in tetralogy of Fallot with pulmonary atresia. A quantitative cineangiographic study. J. Thorac Cardiovasc Surg 1988;95:1045–58.

12. Mair DD, Edwards WD, Julsrud PR, Hagler DJ, Puga FJ. Pulmonary atresia and ventricular septal defect. In: Adams FH, Emmanouilides GC, Riemenschneider TA, editors. Moss' Heart disease in infants, children and adolescents. Baltimore, Hong Kong, London, Sydney: Williams & Wilkins, 4th ed, 1989:289–301.

13. Macartney FJ, Scott O, Deverall PB. Hemodynamic and anatomical characteristics of pulmonary blood supply in pulmonary atresia with ventricular spetal defect. Including a case of persistent fifth aortic arch. Br Heart J 1974;36:1049–61.

14. Lafargue RT, Vogel JHT, Pryor R, Blount SG Jr. Pseudo truncus arteriosus. A review of 21 cases with observations on the oldest reported case. Am J. Cardiol 1967;19:239–46.

15. Millican JS, Puga FJ, Danielson GK, Schaff HV, Julsrud PR, Mair DD. Staged surgical repair of pulmonary atresia, ventricular septal defect, and hypoplastic, confluent pulmonary arteries. J Thorac Cardiovasc Surg 1986;91:818–25.

16. Alfieri O, Blackstone EH, Kirklin JW, Pacifico AD, Bargeron LM Jr. Surgical treatment in tetralogy of Fallot with pulmonary atresia. J Thorac Cardiovasc Surg 1978;76:321–5.

17. Kirklin JW, Blackstone EH, Shimazaki Y, et al. Survival, functional status, and reoperations after repair of tetralogy of Fallot with pulmonary atresia. J Thorac Cardiovasc Surg 1988;96:102–16.

18. Shimazaki Y, Tokuan Y, Lio M, et al. Pulmonary artery pressure and resistance late after repair of tetralogy of Fallot with pulmonary atresia. J. Thorac Cardiovasc Surg 1990;100:425–40.

19. Puga FJ, Leoni FE, Julsrud PR, Mair DD. Complete repair of pulmonary atresia, ventricular septal defect and severe arborisation anomalies of the central pulmonary arteries. Experience with preliminary unifocalisation procedures in 38 patients. J Thorac Cardiovasc Surg 1989;98:1018–29.

20. Garson A Jr, McNamara DG, Cooley DA. Tetralogy of Fallot. In: Roberts WC, editor. Adult congenital heart disease. Philadelphia: FA Davis Company, 1987:493–519.

8. The Fontan circulation

JOHN HESS

Since Fontan and Baudet described the first case of surgical correction of tricuspid atresia in 1971 [1], the outlook of patients with this cardiac malformation changed dramatically. Since then, the number of patients that underwent this type of surgery increased strongly. The principle of this procedure consists of a bypass of the right ventricle by the creation of a communication between the right atrium and the pulmonary artery. Today various modifications of the original procedure are applied not only to treat tricuspid atresia, but also a wide spectrum of complex cyanotic congenital heart disease [2–4].

Although the surgical repair must be tailored to suit the individual patient, several types of Fontan procedures should be briefly discussed at this place.

Atriopulmonary connections are currently the most widely used type of procedure. These can be established by either direct anastomosis or by insertion of a conduit between the systemic venous atrium (right atrium) and the pulmonary artery system. Direct anastomoses can be constructed either anterior (using the right atrial appendage) or posterior to the aorta. In selected cases the native pulmonary valve can be incorporated into an anterior connection, the so-called Kreutzer procedure [5]. In older patients, a homograft or a bioprosthetic valve may have been incorporated in either direct or conduit connections, independent of their location [6]. Following these atriopulmonary connections the systemic venous blood enters the pulmonary artery system directly, that is without a pumping chamber.

The second group of procedures to be considered are those in which a communication between the right atrial chamber and the (rudimentary) right ventricle is established. Such procedures generally are only applicable in patients with tricuspid atresia and normally related great vessels. The communication is established either by a direct anastomosis of the right atrial appendage to the subpulmonary outlet chamber, or by insertion of a valved or

John Hess and George R. Sutherland (eds.), Congenital Heart Disease in Adolescents and Adults, 117–123.
© 1992 *Kluwer Academic Publishers. Printed in the Netherlands.*

non-valved conduit [7]. Although the incorporation of a ventricular chamber may be beneficial to drive pulmonary blood flow, in clinical experience there has been little evidence that these procedures are advantageous over atriopulmonary connections.

Recently these two principal groups of procedures have been extended by further approach which is termed total cavopulmonary connection [8]. A prosthetic patch is sutured into the right atrial cavity so as to produce an intracardiac channel to direct inferior caval venous blood to the pulmonary artery. The superior caval vein is anastomosed to the right pulmonary artery in an end-to-side fashion. Since its introduction in 1988, this procedure has been shown to be applicable to a range of patients with complex congenital heart disease other than tricuspid atresia. In addition, further modifications have been developed. The most important one includes fenestration of the prosthetic patch, which allows for controlled right-to-left shunting in patients with border-line pulmonary vascular resistance. This procedure is often referred to as 'fenestrated Fontan'. The baffle fenestration is subsequently closed once the patient is completely stabilized.

Before the introduction of the Fontan concept in the repair of tricuspid atresia, a superior vena cava to pulmonary artery end-to-end anastomosis was designed by Glenn for palliation of a range of cyanotic congenital cardiac defects including the univentricular heart. These shunts provided adequate palliation in a large number of patients, however the frequent development of arteriovenous fistulas resulted in a dramatic decrease in the use of this approach [9]. With the introduction of the bidirectional cavopulmonary shunt, that is an end-to-side anastomosis between the superior caval vein and the right pulmonary artery, there is now a renewed interest in this technique [8, 10]. This latter shunt constitutes an integral part in the creation of a total cavopulmonary connection.

The initial concept of the Fontan circulation was related to variables such as atrial contractility, the presence of sinus rhythm, pulmonary vascular resistance and pulmonary vascular dimensions and patient's age [1, 10]. This was based upon the fact that in the absence of a pumping ventricle, the major driving force for antegrade pulmonary blood flow originated from the right atrium, which should be qualified for this. A two to three fold rise in right atrial pressure occurred in these patients to supply adequate pulmonary blood flow. This elevated right atrial pressure proved to be one of the crucial determinants of the Fontan circulation. However, this was also the source for concern on the long term performance of these patients. More in particularly, the effects of chronic elevated central venous pressure on liver- and kidney function, as described in patients with chronic right heart failure, were the subject of many studies performed in these patients [7, 10–14].

Although concern is still present, may be even more than twenty years ago, the original concepts have been changed. This is partly due to more sophisticated diagnostic and surgical techniques, partly to more insight into the variables that determine the Fontan circulation.

Changing concept of the Fontan circulation

Today, we know that the Fontan circulation is feasible in case of direct intra-atrial inferior caval vein-pulmonary artery connections, without any support from the side of atrial contraction. Pulsed wave doppler evaluation of pulmonary artery blood flow demonstrates that the flow pattern changes only little during the cardiac cycle. However, major variations are found with respiration. Forward flow decreases with expiration and peaks during inspiration. Similar flow patterns can be demonstrated in patients with Glenn shunts when the pulse wave Doppler sampling volume is placed within the pulmonary artery, distal to the shunt [12].

The original claim that atrial contractility or atrial wall thickness is of crucial importance for maintaining pulmonary circulation seems therefore not justified. In view of this a similar argument seems to be present related to the existence of sinus rhythm. If right atrial contraction does not play a major role in the augmentation of pulmonary bloodflow, the presence of sinus rhythm is not important. However, in Fontan patients not having sinus rhythm the cardiac performance is definitely decreased. Another striking feature is the fact, that in Fontan patients the cardiac output is decreased, both at rest and at exercise, sometimes far below normal levels. These aspects raise the question which major factors determine the circulation after a Fontan procedure, especially in those patients in whom a right ventricle is not incorporated in the Fontan connection.

Of course a low pulmonary vascular resistance is a condition sine qua non, since major right sided forces to augment pulmonary blood flow are not present. Furthermore, pulmonary venous return must be absolutely unobstructed as the compliance of the left ventricle. Since flows, pressures and resistances are ranged on very low levels, even minor changes in these variables may cause serious circulatory impairement. In this view emphasis on left ventricular compliance has only been made more recently [10, 13, 15]. Since important right sided driving forces are frequently absent and pulmonary venous return unobstructed, left ventricular compliance and performance probably are the crucial determinants of the Fontan circulation. Relaxation and upward movement of the ventricle enhances pulmonary blood flow as can be demonstrated by pulsed wave Doppler evaluation of pulmonary venous flow [15, 16]. Following left atrial contraction there is some degree of reversed flow. Forward flow occurs with a biphasic flow pattern, the larger peak most often occurring during ventricular systole. In case of irregular rhythm pulmonary venous flow patterns are highly variable and reflect the incoordinate interaction between the left atrial and ventricular chamber. This is even more so during 'badly timed' closure of the mitral valve, when systolic venous flow is reversed. Therefore, sinus rhythm is very important for maintaining adequate circulation in Fontan patients.

In many patients there has been left ventricular volume overload before the Fontan procedure, in others relative myocardial ischaemia due to hypoxaemia.

Both factors are related to impaired left ventricular function, especially if these factors existed for a long time. This may be a strong argument in favour of early Fontan procedures, as has been proven to be feasible by different groups. Does this aspect explain the low cardiac output in Fontan patients? It has been demonstrated both clinically and in experimental studies, that the left ventricle performs on a low level [10, 13, 14, 17, 18]. Ejection fraction, Vmax and dp/dt are generally significantly related to coronary blood flow, that proved to be impaired due to a relative obstruction to coronary venous return, caused by elevated mean right atrial pressure. Detour of the coronary sinus to the systemic part of the circulation, as is the case in direct intra-atrial inferior caval vein-pulmonary artery connection, will improve coronary blood flow and thus left ventricular function. However, this implicates right-to-left shunting. More insight into the specific aspects of this pattern is needed.

Follow-up of Fontan patients for assessment of cardiac function and specific sequelae

Although the early and late results of Fontan-type procedures have improved considerably over the past decade, a large proportion of these patients will have residual or acquired hemodynamic lesions. Whereas some of these lesions are residual from suboptimal surgical repair, others may develop during the late follow-up and may lead to either acute or progressive clinical deterioration. The clinical manifestation of these problems are not always presented by circulatory signs, but also by non-cardiac symptoms such as protein-losing enteropathy and thrombosis. Therefore a close follow-up of all patients who underwent a Fontan-type procedure is required.

As mentioned before, Fontan patients generally have a decreased cardiac output and a diminished exercise performance, even in the absence of residual morphological or functional lesions. As a consequence of this, the oxygen transport capacity is increased by a rise in hemoglobin concentration. This may lead to polycythaemia. This, in combination with slow flow patterns in the right heart, may give rise to right atrial thrombus formation. However, in the majority of cases this will be associated with a recent history of atrial fibrillation, obstruction to pulmonary blood flow or both [19–21]. Recently, thrombotic lesions, also in the systemic circulation, have been associated with a significant incidence of decreased levels of coagulation proteins in Fontan patients [11]. More particularly, protein S and protein C concentrations in serum of Fontan patients prove to be decreased in about 50%. This phenomenon seems not to be related to liver dysfunction or to the level of central venous pressures. Although the exact mechanism is unknown yet, concern and special attention for this complication seems to be indicated. It is our policy to recommend to patients with this feature anti-thrombotic regimens during certain circumstances, such as immobilization, extra-cardiac surgery, etc.

Persistent arterial desaturation following a Fontan-type procedure is a frequent finding [17]. In the majority of cases this will be caused by a residual communication between the atrial chambers at the site of the former atrial septal defect, or by multiple leaks at the suture line of the patch used for total cavopulmonary connection. In the presence of the elevated right atrial pressures a continuous right-to-left atrial shunt results, which increases in magnitude during exercise. In patients with double inlet left ventricle, in whom the right sided atrioventricular valve has been closed incompletely at the time of the Fontan procedure, persistent arterial desaturation may be present due to diastolic right atrium to left ventricle shunting. In these patients a left-to-right shunt will occur during systole.

Echocardiography, especially by the transoesophageal route, has been shown to be the diagnostic tool of choice in these patients [15]. Rapid recognition and quantification of this complication is indicated for an adequate therapeutic approach. Reoperation has been proven to be successful in the majority of patients. Recently, transcatheter device closure of this defects have been reported and it may be expected that this therapeutic approach may become the technique of first choice.

Obstruction to pulmonary blood flow may either be present in the immediate postoperative period or may be a slowly progressive lesion in the late follow-up, which ultimately requires reoperation [21]. In particular, longstanding Dacron conduits, and bioprosthetic valves incorporated in atriopulmonary connections are at high risk to become obstructed over the longterm follow-up period. Progressive calcification, pronounced neo-intimal thickening and non-pulsatile bloodflow are among the underlying factors. The clinical presentation of this complication may vary. Some patients present with chronic or progressive exercise intolerance and chronic heart failure, some present with more or less isolated atrial dysrhythmia. This latter presentation should be emphasized. All Fontan patients with so called isolated supraventricular dysrhythmia need careful assessment of the structural and functional cardiac status before treatment is initiated. We were frequently faced with patients being on anti-arhythmic drug medication because of atrial fibrillation, that proved to be caused by an obstruction in the Fontan connection.

Proper assessment of obstruction to pulmonary bloodflow is difficult. Since right heart and pulmonary artery pressures are low, even intracardiac pressure measurements may underestimate the severity of obstruction. Both angiocardiography and echocardiography may be of great value, however, sometimes only imaging by means of magnetic resonance may assess the morphological aspects adequately.

Although obstruction to pulmonary blood flow and atrial thrombus formation are among the most serious immediate or long-term hemodynamic sequelae following Fontan-type procedures, a range of other hemodynamic lesions may be encountered which impair functional capacity and may require either early or late reoperation.

Atrioventricular valve incompetence is frequently found following Fontan procedures. In particular, in patients who were operated at an older age the longstanding left ventricular overload may result in annular dilatation with resultant atrioventricular valve regurgitation. In those patients with complex cardiac lesions, such as common atrioventricular valves or univentricular hearts, atrioventricular valve regurgitation is frequently encountered already preoperatively. Valve replacement in the Fontan situation must be avoided at all costs, since it inevitably increases left atrial pressures and therefore the afterload of the pulmonary circulation. Consequently this is followed by a further rise in right atrial pressures and a likely decrease in cardiac output.

Obstruction to the systemic circulation is a further complication that may occur in patients with discordant ventriculo-arterial connections, with the aorta arising from a rudimentary outlet chamber, in whom the ventricular septal defect may become restrictive [10]. Even relatively small gradients across the ventricular septal defect may impair ventricular compliance and therefore increase the afterload of the pulmonary circulation. The effect of elevated right atrial pressure itself may give rise to specific problems both early and late postoperatively. Pericardial effusions and pleural effusions may occur shortly after surgery and are sometimes difficult to treat. However, these complications may also occur at late follow-up and are then frequently related to impaired cardiac function and a further increase in right atrial pressure. Also in these situations examination for underlying problems such as thrombi, obstruction to pulmonary bloodflow and impaired ventricular function is indicated.

Protein losing enteropathy may occur both early and late postoperatively resulting in hypoalbuminaemia and generalized oedema [22]. Intravascular volume may be decreased, leading to a too low preload for the pulmonary circulation. The protein loss has been associated with intestinal lymfangiectasia due to elevated venous pressure. Dietary recommendations and diuretic treatment may relieve symptoms, although structural management is only seldomly possible.

Regular evaluation of patients after Fontan procedures, even in the absence of symptoms, is necessary to achieve the best quality of life. Early recognition of problems as mentioned above can only be done if adequate knowledge of both diagnostic and therapeutic aspects is available. Experience with rather confessional diagnostic tools, such as cardiac catheterization and transthoracic echocardiography has proven to be insufficient to deal with this group of patients. Newer techniques, such as transoesophageal echocardiography and magnetic resonance imaging must be available and interpretable. In case of managing adult patients close collaboration with pediatric cardiologists is necessary to maintain the understanding of the changing concepts on the clinics and pathophysiology of the Fontan circulation.

References

1. Fontan F, Baudet E. Surgical repair of tricuspid atresia. Thorax 1871;26:240–8.
2. DeLeon SY, Ilbawi MN, Idriss FS, et al. Fontan type operation for complex lesions – Surgical considerations to improve survival. J Thorac Cardiovasc Surg 1986;92:1029–37.
3. Stellin G, Mazzucco A, Bortolotti U, et al. Tricuspid atresia versus other complex lesions. J Thorac Cardiovasc Surg 1988;96:204–11.
4. Mayer JE, Helgason H, Jonas RA, et al. Extending the limits for modified Fontan procedures. J Thorac Cardiovasc Surg 1986;92:1021–8.
5. Kreutzer GO, Vargas FJ, Schlichter AJ, et al. Atriopulmonary anastomosis. J. Thorac Cardiovasc Surg 1982;83:427–36.
6. Eijgelaar A, Hess J, Hardjowijno R, Karliczek GF, Rating W, Homan vd Heide JN. Experience with the Fontan operation. Thorac Cardiovasc Surg 1982;30:63–8.
7. Coles JG, Leung M, Kielmanowicz, et al. Repair of tricuspid atresia: Utility of right ventricular incorporation. Ann Thorac Surg 1988;45:384–9.
8. DeLeval MR, Kilner P, Gewillig M, Bull C. Total cavopulmonary connection: A logical alternative to atriopulmonary connection for complex Fontan operations. Experimental studies and early clinical experience. J Thorac Cardiovasc Surg 1988;96:682–95.
9. Bargeron LM, Karp RB, Barcia A. Kirklin JW, Hunt D, Deverall PB. Late deterioration of patients after superior vena cava to ribht pulmonary artery anastomosis. Am J Cardiol 1972;30:211–6.
10. Fontan F, Kirklin JW, Fernandez G, et al. Outcome after a 'perfect' Fontan operation. Circulation 1990;81:1520–36.
11. Cromme-Dijkhuis AH, Henkens CMA, Bijleveld CMA, Hillige HL, Bom VJJ, vd Meer J. Coagulation factor abnormalities as possible risk factor after Fontan operations. Lancet 1990;336:1087–90.
12. Disessa TG, Child JS, Perloff JK, et al. Systemic venous and pulmonary arterial flow patterns after Fontan's procedure for tricuspid atresia or single ventricle. Circulation 1984;70:898–902.
13. Gewillig HM, Lundström UR, Bull C, Wyse RKH, Deanfield JE. Exercise response in patients with congenital heart disease after Fontan repair: Patterns and determinants of performance. J Am Coll Cardiol 1990;15:1424–32.
14. Girod DA, Fontan F, Deville C, Ottenkamp J, Choussat A. Long-term results after the Fontan operation for tricuspid atresia. Circulation 1987;75:605–10.
15. Stümper O, Sutherland GR, Geuskens R, Roelandt JRTC, Bos E, Hess J. Transesophageal echocardiography in the evaluation and management of the Fontan circulation. J Am Coll Cardiol 1991;17:1152–60.
16. Hagler DJ, Seward JB, Tajik AJ, Ritter DG. Functional assessment of the Fontan operation: Combined M-mode, two-dimensional and Doppler echocardiographic studies. J Am Coll Cardiol 1984;4:756–64.
17. Leung MP, Benson LN, Smallhorn JF, Williams WG, Trusler GA, Freedom RM. Abnormal cardiac signs after Fontan type of operation: indicators of residua and sequelae. Br Heart J 1989;61:52–8.
18. Matsuda H, Kawashima Y, Takano H, Miyamoto K, Mori T. Experimental evaluation of atrial function in right atrium-pulmonary artery conduit operations for tricuspid atresia. J Thorac Cardiovasc Surg 1981;81:762–7.
19. Dobell ARC, Trusler GA, Smallhorn JF, Williams WG. Atrial thrombi formation after the Fontan operation. Ann Thorac Surg 1986;42:664–7.
20. Nakazawa M, Nakanishi T, Okuda H, et al. Dynamics of right heart flow patterns in patients after Fontan procedure. Circulation 1984;69:306–12.
21. Fernandez G, Costa F, Fontan F, Naftel DC, Blackstone EH, Kirklin JW. Prevalence of reoperation for pathway obstruction after the Fontan operation. Ann Thorac Surg 1989;48:654–9.
22. Hess J, Kruizinga K, Bijleveld CMA, Hardjowijono R,k Eygelaar A. Protein-losing enteropathy after Fontan operation. J Thorac Cardiovasc Surg 1984;88:606–9.

9. Non-invasive assessment of the Fontan circulation

LIV HATLE

Introduction

The Fontan procedure was first used in tricuspid atresia, and with modifications of the technique its use has been extended to single ventricles and various other complex congenital lesions [1–3]. Following the Fontan procedure blood flow into the pulmonary artery is through a direct connection from the right atrium or right atrial appendage to the main pulmonary artery. Modifications of the procedure include direct connections from the systemic veins to the pulmonary artery with extracardial or intraatrial conduits, or including a hypoplastic right ventricle in the connection to the pulmonary artery, with or without a valve.

Noninvasive assessment of the circulation following this operation includes visualization of the chambers, great vessels and connections with two-dimensional echocardiography, and recording of the blood flow velocities within these structures with Doppler [4, 5]. This can be achieved by transthoracic imaging in many patients, but added information, especially about posterior structures, can be obtained by transesophageal echocardiography [6] and thrombi and conduit obstructions can be diagnosed. Two-dimensional (color-coded) Doppler can be helpful in detecting residual leaks. With these techniques the functional result of the procedure can be assessed. In addition, by comparing the flow velocity curves in the pulmonary artery with those in the systemic and pulmonary veins and across the systemic atrio-ventricular valve, information can be obtained about the mechanisms influencing forward flow into the pulmonary artery in the Fontan circulation. Information about the circulation through the lungs can be obtained by ventilation and perfusion scintigraphy [7, 8].

John Hess and George R. Sutherland (eds.), Congenital Heart Disease in Adolescents and Adults, 125–132.
© *1992 Kluwer Academic Publishers. Printed in the Netherlands.*

Determinants of pulmonary artery flow in the Fontan circulation

In the absence of right ventricular pump function, the systolic function of the right atrium has been considered important. Several studies have shown that atrial contraction results in increased velocity of flow into the pulmonary artery [9–11]. Sinus rythm was initially one of the criteria in selecting patients for this procedure, but satisfactory long term clinical results have been shown also in patients without sinus rhythm [12].

In most patients a biphasic velocity pattern is described [4–6, 9–11], in addition onset of forward flow prior to atrial contraction has been noted [5]. The mechanism causing the second peak has not been clearly shown although left heart events have been suggested.

Changes in intrathoracic pressure with respiration may also contribute to forward flow, and marked increases in forward flow velocity during inspiration can be seen in some patients [6].

Relation between pulmonary artery, systemic and pulmonary vein velocities

Figure 1 shows a recording from the pulmonary artery in a patient with a right atrial- to- pulmonary artery connection. Forward flow is triphasic and with

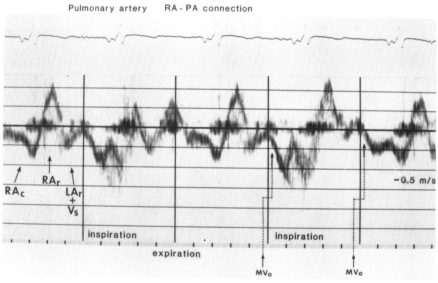

Figure 1. The flow velocity in the pulmonary artery recorded in a patient with a right atrial-to-pulmonary artery (RA-PA) connection. Forward flow is away from the transducer, it is triphasic with increase in forward flow following right atrial contraction (RAc). This is followed by flow reversal, likely due to right atrial relaxation (RAr). The forward flow in late systole may be due to left atrial relaxation (LAr) and ventricular systole (Vs), and in a diastole increase in forward flow follows shortly after mitral valve opening (MVo) as indicated by vertical arrows. Increase in forward flow velocity with inspiration is also seen.

inspiratory increase in velocity. At atrial contraction increase in forward flow velocity is seen, and this is followed by flow reversal, likely due to right atrial relaxation. Following this reversal there is forward flow during late systole, decreasing toward endsystole. In diastole forward flow prior to atrial contraction is seen. As indicated in Figure 1 the forward flow in late systole and in early diastole may be attributed to left heart events. By comparing pulmonary artery and mitral flow velocities it can be shown that the early diastolic increase in velocity in the pulmonary artery regularly starts 80–100 ms after mitral valve opening. It is therefore likely caused by the decrease in ventricular and left atrial pressure in early diastole, with this pressure decrease transmitted through the pulmonary circulation and, with a slight time delay, resulting in forward flow into a pulmonary artery. The forward flow seen in late systole could, in a similar way, result from the decrease in left atrial pressure during systole, due to left atrial relaxation as well as to ventricular systole.

In Figure 2 the relation between the flow velocities in the pulmonary artery and in the hepatic and pulmonary veins can be seen. Right atrial contraction results in forward flow in the pulmonary artery and at the same time reversal into the hepatic vein. Right atrial relaxation has the opposite result, with forward flow in the hepatic vein and reversal in the pulmonary artery. On the other hand, the forward flow in late systole and early diastole are of the same direction in both vessels, only with a later onset in the hepatic vein, again suggesting that they are both due to left heart events.

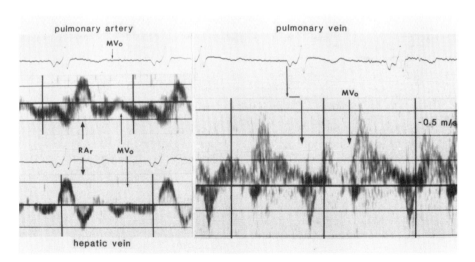

Figure 2. Comparison between pulmonary artery and hepatic vein velocities shows opposite direction of flow at right atrial contraction as well as relaxation (RAr), while in late systole and early diastole flow direction is similar in the two vessels, but with a delay in the hepatic vein. In the pulmonary vein flow reversal following atrial contraction is seen, forward flow velocity in systole is reduced with increase following mitral valve opening (MVo).

The pulmonary vein shows reversal of flow with atrial contraction, followed by forward flow in systole and again at the time of mitral valve opening. This velocity pattern is normal except for a slight reduction in velocity of forward flow in systole. From the onset of this systolic flow it can be seen that left atrial relaxation starts a little later than on the right side. In the pulmonary artery both the systolic and early diastolic forward flow seem to have the same time delay compared to forward flow in the pulmonary vein.

This suggested relationship between left heart pressure changes and forward flow in the pulmonary artery is supported by findings in patients with atrial arrhythmias. In Figure 3 atrial contractions are seen to occur during systole, resulting in cannon waves in the pulmonary vein. With the same rhythm a similar reversal is seen in the pulmonary artery, only with a slight delay compared to the cannon wave in the pulmonary vein. The patient had a direct caval-pulmonary artery shunt without right atrial contractions influencing flow into the pulmonary artery, indicating that the reversals represent the cannon waves transmitted through the pulmonary circulation from the left heart. In this situation forward flow velocity in the pulmonary artery is also more similar to that in the pulmonary vein, suggesting that the pulsatile flow is determined by left heart events, only with the exception of the inspiratory increase which occurs earlier and is better seen in the pulmonary artery.

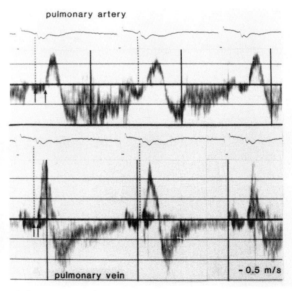

Figure 3. Forward flow is away from the transducer both in the pulmonary vein and the pulmonary artery, and atrial contractions during systole result in marked flow reversal in the pulmonary vein (cannon waves). Similar reversals are also seen in the pulmonary artery, these occur a little later and are likely transmitted from the left side, since the patient had a direct caval-pulmonary artery shunt. Note similarity between the pulmonary vein and pulmonary artery flow when there is a direct venoarterial connection.

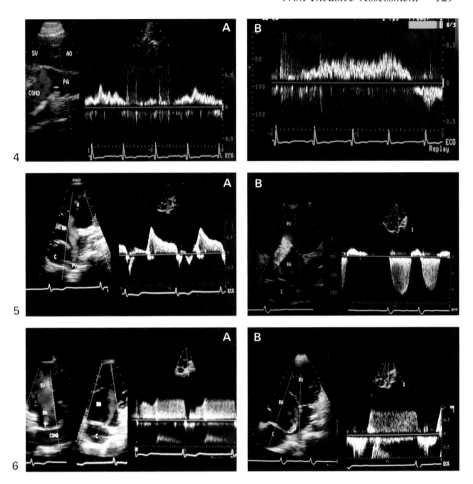

Figure 4. A: is recorded from the connection between the conduit (cond) from the inferior caval vein to the pulmonary artery (PA). Flow is toward the transducer, pulsatile and with marked respiratory variation. AO – aorta, SV – single ventricle. B: is recorded during deeper respiration and shows more increase in forward flow velocity, but also reversal of flow at expiration.

Figure 5. A: shows the flow from the pulmonary vein (PV) into the atrium (RA) and ventricle (V). The pulsed Doppler recording from the pulmonary vein shows mainly diastolic filling, systolic filling is markedly reduced with the slight reversals at beginning and end-systole. C-conduit. B: shows the A-V valve regurgitation in another patient, the CW Doppler recording shows a reduced rate of rise of the regurgitant velocity. RV-systemic ventricle, RA-pulmonary venous atrium, C-conduit.

Figure 6. A: The 2D recording shows two small leaks from the conduit to the pulmonary venous atrium. The pulsed Doppler recording shows continuous shunting, with some reduction in velocity in systole. The velocity indicates that the pressure in the conduit is 4–5 mmHg higher than in the pulmonary venous atrium. B: is recorded from the patient shown in Fig. 5B, there is a small leak from the conduit with right to left shunting throughout diastole, but with reversal in systole due to pressure increase in the atrium due to significant regurgitation.

When the right atrium is excluded from the veno-pulmonary artery connection, the increase in forward pulmonary flow at atrial contraction will no longer be seen, and in the absence of cannon waves and severe A-V valve regurgitation, flow reversals both in the pulmonary artery and in the systemic veins is mainly influenced by respiration, occuring on expiration. In Figure 4A both the pulsatility of flow in a conduit from the inferior vena cava to the pulmonary artery and a marked respiratory variation can be seen, with little or no forward flow during expiration. With deeper respiration (Figure 4B) the inspiratory increase in flow is more marked, but in addition flow reversal on expiration is seen.

Forward flow in the pulmonary artery can therefore be influenced by right atrial function and by respiration, as well as by left heart events that influence left atrial filling, such as ventricular function and atrioventricular valve regurgitation.

Ventricular function/A-V valve regurgitation

Pulmonary venous flow is influenced by left atrial function [13]. Ventricular function is another important determinant of pulmonary venous flow. The systolic function influences left atrial filling by the degree of downward annular motion [14]. This may be assessed by two-dimensional and M-mode echocardiography. Information about systolic function may also be obtained from the rate of increase of the velocity of A-V valve regurgitation.

Abnormal diastolic function due to hypertrophy may result in reduced early diastolic filling. Decrease in ventricular compliance may result in higher diastolic pressures and more early diastolic filling. Such changes may be assessed from the forward flow across the atrio-ventricular valve and forward as well as reverse flow in the pulmonary veins. Both systolic and diastolic dysfunction as well as regurgitation in the systemic A-V valve may result in increased left atrial pressure, and this will influence left atrial filling and the velocity of flow in the pulmonary vein. In Figure 5A the systolic filling is reduced, probably due to a combined effect of reduced ventricular function and moderate A-V valve regurgitation.

Regurgitations are easily diagnosed and semiquantitation is possible, partly from the width of the beginning of the regurgitant jet. Figure 5B is recorded from a patient with significant A-V valve regurgitation, which resulted in systolic flow reversal in the pulmonary vein.

Reduced ventricular function as well as significant A-V valve regurgitation may therefore, in addition to possible increases in pulmonary vascular resistance and conduit obstruction, be of importance for the potential complications that may be seen following the Fontan procedure due to low flow and high venous pressures.

Atrial arrhythmias

The presence of atrial arrhythmias may result in reduction in forward flow, due to loss of left, as well as right, atrial function, and/or a shortened filling time at rapid heart rates, and to left atrial cannon waves.

Atrial tachyarrhythnias may result in marked decreases in exercise tolerance or increase in symptoms.

Residual shunts

The presence of residual shunts may be diagnosed with two-dimensional color-coded Doppler as shown in Figure 6. Posteriorly located leaks may be more easily detected from the esophagus. The presence of leaks gives the possibility to obtain the pressure difference between the systemic veins and the pulmonary venous atrium. The marked difference in shunt velocity between diastole and systole seen in Figure 6B, indicates the marked rise in atrial pressure due to significant A-V valve regurgitation. Intrapulmonary shunts are not visualized by Doppler, but may be diagnosed by contrast echocardiography and diagnosed as well as assessed by ventilation and perfusion scintigraphy [7, 8].

Conduit obstruction

Deterioration of function may be due to obstruction of the conduit due to thrombi or obstruction at the site of the anastomosis. Thrombi are more likely to be detected by transesophageal imaging [6]. Obstructions may be diagnosed by imaging or by recording abnormal flow by color or conventional pulsed Doppler. This may be detected by the transthoracic approach, but more likely from the esophagus, especially for posterior structures [6].

Cardiac output, exercise studies

Cardiac output can be obtained noninvasively by recording the diameter of the aortic annulus and the flow velocity integral across the annulus. If there is more than mild aortic regurgitation, stroke volume and cardiac output will be overestimated. The flow velocity in the ascending aorta can also be recorded during exercise, making it possible to assess changes in stroke volume and cardiac output with exercise [15].

Conclusion

With combined two-dimensional imaging and Doppler from a transthoracic or transesophageal approach both anatomy and flow can be assessed. Flow into the pulmonary artery in the Fontan circulation is, in addition to the effect of right atrial contraction and of respiration, markedly influenced by the systemic ventricle, atrium and A-V valve function. Preoperative ventricular function is therefore likely to be of importance for the Fontan circulation, along with pulmonary vascular resistance and the size of the pulmonary artery at surgery [10].

References

1. Fontan F, Baudet E. Surgical repair of tricuspid atresia. Thorax 1971;26:240–8.
2. Gale AW, Danielson GK, McGoon DC, Mair DD. Modified Fontan operation for univentricular heart and complicated congenital lesions. J Thorac Cardiovasc Surg 1979;78:831–8.
3. Kawashima Y, Kitamura S, Matsuda H, Shimazaki Y, Nakano S, Hirose H. Total cavopulmonary shunt operation in complex cardiac anomalies. J Thorac Cardiovasc Surg 1984;87:74.
4. Hagler DJ, Seward JB, Tajik AJ, Ritter DG. Functional assessment of the Fontan operation: Combined M–mode, two–dimensional and Doppler echocardiographic studies. J Am Coll Cardiol 1984;4:756–64.
5. DiSessa TG, Child JS, Perloff JK, et al. Systemic venous and pulmonary arterial flow patterns after Fontans procedure for tricuspid atresia or single ventricle. Circulation 1987;70:898–902.
6. Stümper O, Sutherland GR, Geuskens R, Roelandt JRTC, Bos E, Hess J. Transesophageal echocardiography in evaluation and management after a Fontan procedure. J Am Coll Cardiol 1991;17:1152–60.
7. Cloutier A, Ash JM, Smallhorn JF, et al. Abnormal distribution of pulmonary blod flow after the Glenn shunt or Fontan procedure: Risk of development of arteriovenous fistulae. Circulation 1985;72:471–9.
8. Matsushita T, Matsuda H, Ogawa M, et al. Assessment of the intrapulmonary ventilation–perfusion distribution after the Fontan procedure for complex cardiac anomalies: Relation to pulmonary hemodynamics. J AM Coll Cardiol 1990;15:842–8.
9. Nakazawa M, Nakanishi T, Okuda H, et al. Dynamics of right heart flow in patients after Fontan procedure. Circulation 1984;69:306–12.
10. Nakazawa M, Nojima K, Okuda H, et al. Flow dynamics in the main pulmonary artery after the Fontan procedure in patients with tricuspid atresia or single ventricle. Circulation 1987;75:1117–23.
11. Qureshi SA, Richheimer R, McKay R, Arnold R. Doppler echocardiographic evaluation of pulmonary artery flow after modified Fontan operation: Importance of atrial contraction. Br Heart J 1990;64:272–6.
12. Alboliras ET, Porter CJ, Danielson GK, et al. Results of the modified Fontan operation for congenital heart lesions in patients without preoperative sinus rhythm. J Am Coll Cardiol 1985;6:228–33.
13. Keren G, Bier A, Sherez J, Miura D, Keefe D, LeJemtel T. Atrial contraction is an important determinant of pulmonary venous flow. J Am Coll Cardiol 1986;7:693–5.
14. Keren G, Sonnenblick EH, LeJemtel TH. Mitral annulus motion. Relation to pulmonary venous and transmitral flows in normal subjects and in patients with dilated cardiomyopathy. Circulation 1988;78:1–9.
15. Gewillig MH, Lundstrøm UR, Bull C, Wyse RKH, Deanfield JE. Exercise responses in patients with congenital heart disease after Fontan repair: Patterns and determinants of performance. J Am Col Cardiol 1990;15:1424–32.

10. Supraventricular arrhythmias in congenital heart disease

MARGREET TH.E. BINK-BOELKENS

Supraventricular arrhythmias may occur in adolescents with unoperated or inoperable congenital heart disease, but are more frequent in adolescents who underwent cardiac surgery. These arrhythmias may be present in the early postoperative period, which is beyond the scope of this chapter, but often develop in the years after surgery. Usually there is no relation between the hemodynamic result of the operation and the presence or absence of arrhythmias. This contrasts with the unoperated group, in which hemodynamic problems often lead to the development of supraventricular arrhythmias. Although the supraventricular arrhythmias are usually well tolerated, they can cause morbidity and even mortality.

Etiology

The supraventricular part of the conduction system consists of the sinus node, the three atrial preferential pathways and the atrioventricular node. The arterial blood supply of the sinus node is very variable; in 55 percent it is a branch of the right coronary artery and in 45 percent of the left coronary artery. The sinus node artery runs either clockwise or counter-clockwise around the superior vena cava [1]. Moreover, the different congenital heart malformations have their specific patterns of blood supply to the sinus node [2–4]. Blood supply to the atrioventricular mode is through a terminal branch of the right coronary artery (90 percent).

In unoperated and inoperable congenital heart disease, abnormal pressure or volume load can result in atrial dilatation and stretch of the atrial wall and the adjacent conduction tissue. This changes the sinus and atrioventricular node function and the automaticity of the atrial myocardium. In addition cyanosis and dilatation poduce fibrosis of the atrial wall, a substrate for reentrant tachycardias [5].

133

John Hess and George R. Sutherland (eds.), Congenital Heart Disease in Adolescents and Adults, 133–145.
© 1992 *Kluwer Academic Publishers. Printed in the Netherlands.*

During surgery in the atrium, all parts of the conduction system are at risk. The sinus node may be damaged during cannulation of the superior vena cava and by suturing in the sinus node area, as in physiologic correction of transposition of the great arteries. The sinus node artery may also be injured during these pocedures. This artery is especially at risk when its course is partially intra-myocardial or if it originates as a lateral branch of the right coronary artery [3]. An atriotomy, atrial septectomy or an atriopulmonary anastomosis will easily damage the sinus node artery that takes this course. An atriotomy combined with an atrial septectomy may interrupt two or all preferential pathways, often resulting in AVJ rhythm [6]. The atrioventricular node is at risk during suturing in its vicinity but is seldom damaged, probably because its location has been very well defined by the various pathologists [1, 7].

Arrhythmias and electrophysiology

The supraventricular arrhythmias seen in unoperated congenital heart disease are mainly tachy-arrhythmias. After surgery the arrhythmias are brady-arrhythmias (sinus bradycardia, sinus arrest, AVJ rhythm), or tachy-arrhythmias (especially atrial flutter), and more often a combination of brady- and tachy-arrhythmias. Atrial fibrillation is rare in young patients and is mainly seen if the atria are very dilated or as a deterioration of atrial flutter. The atrioventricular node in young people can easily conduct atrial flutter 1:1 during exercise. Therefore, suppression of 1:1 conduction with drugs may be very difficult in this age group.

Electrophysiologic studies in pre-operative ASD patients revealed depressed sinus- and atrioventricular node function [8, 9]. Electrophysiologic studies after Mustard and Fontan operations have shown sinus node dysfunction, intra-atrial conduction delay and dispersion of refractoriness in most patients [10, 11]. Supraventricular tachycardia or atrial flutter could be induced in many patients, facilitated by the inhomogeneous conduction and by anatomic obstacles such as scars and patch material. In these patients cessation of tachycardia often results in severe bradycardia by overdrive suppression of the diseased sinus node, and in turn, severe bradycardia elicits tachycadia [12]. In postoperative patients with atrial flutter the incidence of underlying sinus node disease is high [13, 14]. Cardioversion of atrial flutter can therefore result in severe bradycardia or arrest and should only be performed if back-up pacing is possible.

Unoperated congenital heart disease

Atrial septal defect

The incidence of supraventricular tachycardia, atrial fibrillation and atrial flutter in adults with unoperated ASD is 8–28 percent [15, 16]. Brandenburg et al. [17] found that 70 percent of the patients aged 44 years and older continued to have these arrhythmias after operation. Supraventricular arrhythmias are also seen in 8 percent of children with unoperated ASD, but these are less significant and tend to disappear after surgery at a young age (3–5 yrs.) [9, 18].

Ebstein's Anomaly of the tricuspid valve

In Ebstein's anomaly, at least 36 percent of the patients have arrhythmias, mainly supraventricular tachycardia or atrial flutter or fibrillation. Ten percent has a WPW syndrome [19]. These arrhythmias contribute substantially to the morbidity but also to the mortality in Ebstein's disease and therefore play a role in the decision about surgery.

Inoperable congenital heart disease

This group consists mainly of patients with irreversible pulmonary hypertension and patients with pulmonary atresia with a hypoplastic pulmonary vasculature. Dubrow et al. [20] found that cyanosis prolonged sinoatrial conduction time and atrial refractoriness. Clinically, however sinus node dysfunction or supraventricular arrhythmias are of minor importance. Ventricular arrhythmias could well be a more important cause of syncope or sudden death, as seen in some of these patients. During the end-stage of the disease, tricuspid insufficiency and atrial dilatation can lead to atrial tachy-arrhythmias.

Postoperative congenital heart disease

Atrial septal defect

Although some young patients with ASD have supraventricular arrhythmias preoperatively, these are usually mild and asymptomatic. However, after ASD closure sometimes supraventricular arrhythmias are seen that require drug treatment or pacemaker implantation. ASD surgery is second on the list of preceding surgery in children who need a pacemaker because of sinus node dysfunction [21]. Bharati and Lev [22] found sutures, foreign body reaction and fibrosis in the sinus node area, the preferential pathways and the approaches of the atrioventricular node in 4 patients who died suddenly years after an ASD repair. In a retrospective study of 204 children after ASD repair, we found a 10 percent incidence of symptomatic arrhythmias that required treatment [14]. After a change in cannulation technique to a selective cannulation of the superior vena cava, symptomatic arrythmias were no longer found in a group of 50 consecutively operated children [18]. This suggests that in ASD repair damage to the conduction tissue can be prevented by surgical modifications.

Physiologic correction of transposition of the great arteries

In physiologic correction of transposition of the great arteries, the systemic venous flow is redirected through the atrium to the left ventricle and pulmonary artery. The pulmonary venous flow is redirected to the right ventricle and the aorta. In the Mustard operation, a pericardial or dacron tunnel (baffle) is used to redirect the blood at atrial level (Figure 1). In the Senning procedure the patient's own atrial tissue is used. The electrophysiologic results of both types of operations are comparable. The incidence of brady- and tachy-arrhythmias after this type of operation is high and increases with age [14, 23, 24]. A recent study of Bogaards et al. [25] in 129 Mustard patients, most of whom were in their second decade, showed that the incidence of passive arrhythmias increased from 20 percent in the first postoperative year to

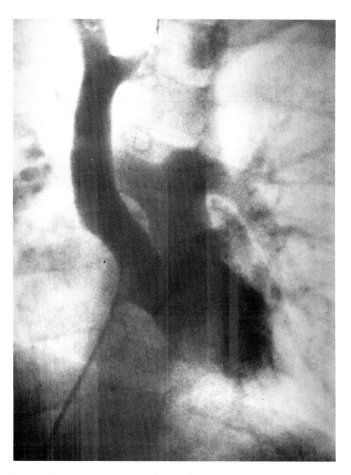

Figure 1. Angiocardiogram after a Mustard operation. The systemic venous flow is redirected to the left ventricle and the pulmonary artery.

65 percent in the 15th year after operation. Similarly the incidence of active arrhythmias (supraventricular tachycardia, atrial flutter) increased from 7 percent to 60 percent in the 18th postoperative year. Sudden death occurs in 4–8 percent of the patients. The major risk factor for sudden death is the presence of atrial flutter [13, 14, 26]. The mechanism leading to sudden death is probably 1:1 conduction of atrial flutter deteriorating into ventricular fibrillation, in view of the fact that many of these children die during exercise, sometimes with a properly functioning pacemaker [14]. Edwards et al. [27] found fibrosis of the sinus node artery and the paranodal tissue in 77–100 percent (depending on the period of follow-up) of children who died after a Mustard operation. Electrophysiologic studies and pathological findings show that damage to the sinus node area inherent in the extensive atrial surgery is responsible for the high incidence of supraventricular arrhythmias [28].

In view of the incidence of supraventricular arrhythmias, the risk of sudden death, the frequent reoperations and the deterioration of right ventricular function with age, anatomic correction of transposition of the great arteries is nowadays preferred to physiologic correction. Mid-term results show a low incidence of supraventricular arrhythmias, no or only mild electrophysiologic abnormalities of the sinus node and no arrhythmia-related sudden death [29–32]. This confirms that supraventricular arrhythmias do not belong to the natural, but to the unnatural history of transposition of the great arteries.

The Fontan operation

The Fontan operation is used in congenital heart disease in which one ventricle is hypoplastic or absent, thus preventing a normal biventricular correction. In the Fontan circulation the normally developed ventricle provides the systemic circulation; the pulmonary circulation is provided by the right atrium, which is connected directly or by a conduit to the pulmonary artery (Figure 2). The consequence of this operation is an elevated right atrial pressure resulting in atrial dilatation. As in preoperative ASD, Ebstein's anomaly and other AV valve abnormalities, this may lead to the development of atrial flutter and atrial tachycardia. As in the physiologic correction of transposition, the sinus node or its artery may be injured during surgery. Battistessa and colleagues [4] found that the sinus node artery originated from the left coronary artery in most hearts with tricuspid atresia. On the way to the sinus node, it crosses the roof of the right atrium to a varying extent. The sinus node artery was found to be damaged in half of the specimens in which a Fontan operation was performed. Therefore, it is not surprising that Kurer et al. [11] found the same electrophysiologic abnormalities after the Fontan operation as Vetter and colleagues [10] after the Mustard operation.

Supraventricular arrhythmias are common after the Fontan operation (Table 1): bradycardia, as well as tachycardia, especially atrial flutter but also atrial tachycardia [33–36]. Porter et al. [35] found a cumulative probability of 42 percent of supraventricular tachy-arrhythmias at a follow-up of 7.5 years. As

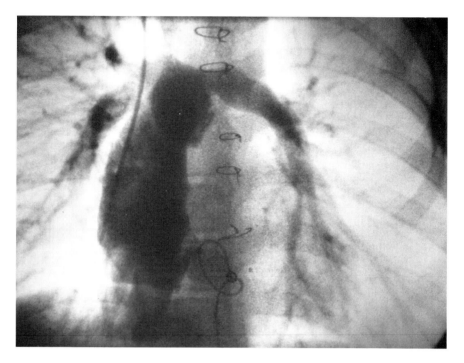

Figure 2. Angiocardiogram after a Fontan operation. The right atrium is directly connected to the pulmonary artery. An epicardial electrode is placed on the ventricle.

Table 1. Late arrhythmias after Fontan operation.

	N	Mean follow-up (yrs)	Brady-cardia	SVT	V.A. $> =$ Lown 4A
Porter [35]	120	7.5	—	37%	—
Chen [34]	24	4.8	22%	35%	22%
Weber [33]	30	6.3	10%	39%	—
Gewillig [36]	78	3.7	0%	14%	0%
Bink[a]	31	6.2	19%	31%	29%

SVT = = Supraventricular tachy-arrhythmias; VA = Ventricular arrhythmias.
[a] = unpublished.

after physiologic correction of transposition of the great arteries, the incidence of arrhythmias increases with length of follow-up [33, 35]. Bradycardia seems less frequent than after the Mustard operation. Acute onset of atrial flutter is sometimes the result of progressive narrowing of the atrio-pulmonary conduit. Late sudden death by arrhythmias is seen after the Fontan operation, but less frequently (3 percent) than after the Mustard operation. In our experience, successful resuscitation of these patients is very difficult, because a good pulmonary flow is seldom obtained by cardiac massage.

For hemodynamic reasons de Leval et al. [37] introduced the total cavopulmonary connection as an alernative for the Fontan operation. The superior vena cava and an intra-atrial tunnel draining the inferior vena cava are directly anastomosed to the right pulmonary artery (Figure 3). Apart from its hemodynamic consequences, this could have a favorable influence on the prevention of arrhythmias, because after this operation the main part of the right atrium is at low pressure. On the other hand, extensive surgery is done in the sinus node area. The results in their first 40 patients show in particular a decrease of early arrhythmias and concomitant mortality [38]. Long-term effects are not yet known.

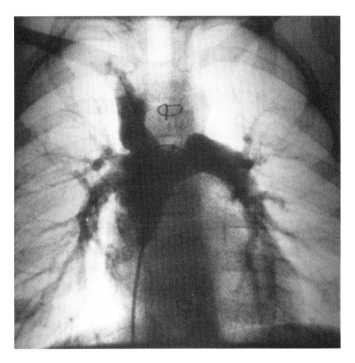

Figure 3. Angiogram from the superior vena cava after a total cavopulmonary connection. The caval veins drain directly into the right pulmonary artery.

Prognosis

The morbidity due to supraventricular arrhythmias in the unoperated group is low. The patients with Ebstein's disease and the Eisenmenger syndrome are an exception. In these patients, arrhythmias lead to increasing cyanosis and depress cardiac function. In the group with operated congenital heart disease the brady-arrhythmias are usually well tolerated. Pediatric cardiologist are often concerned about the low heart rate, but patients seldom have symptoms.

Tachy-arrhythmias more often give symptoms such as palpitations, dizziness, syncope or fatigue. They can also evoke heart failure in patients with a diminished ventricular function, as is so often the case in Fontan patients.

Sudden death by arrhythmias is mainly caused by tachy-arrhythmias, and above all by atrial flutter [13, 14, 26]. The incidence of sudden death also depends on the underlying cardiac status. The highest incidence is seen after the Mustard operation, the lowest after ASD closure. Garson and colleagues [39] published the result of a collaborative study of 380 children with atrial flutter. Eighty percent had previous cardiac surgery. The three most common operations were physiologic correction of transposition (27.6 percent), Blalock Hanlon atrial septectomy (16.1 percent), and ASD closure (11.1 percent). The incidence of sudden death was 5 percent for children with effective control of atrial flutter, but 20 percent in children without effective control, whether or not the ventricular rate was controlled. The mechanism of sudden death seems to be 1:1 conduction of atrial flutter deteriorating into ventricular fibrillation.

Treatment

The indication for treatment of bradycardia is difficult to define in asymptomatic patients with a heart rate that is 'low for their age'. On the other hand, symptoms such as syncope are a clear indication for pacemaker implantation. The same applies to the bradycardic patient who needs to be treated for tachycardia with drugs other than digitalis. The high incidence of sudden death in patients with atrial flutter is the rationale behind a treatment which not only controls ventricular rate, but terminates and prevents atrial flutter at any rate. Treatment often consists of a combination of drug therapy and temporary or permanent pacing. We expect that in the near future surgical and catheter ablation techniques will become increasingly important.

Anti-arrhythmic drugs

Anti-arrhythmic drugs are used to control and to prevent tachycardia. Besides the well-known side effects of drugs there are some specific problems in patients with tachycardia after cardiac surgery. In the first place, many anti-arrhythmic drugs depress sinus node function. Since many patients with tachycardia have underlying sinus node disease, digitalis is often the only drug that can safely be prescribed without pacemaker implantation. Secondly, some drugs have pro-arrhythmic effects. This has recently been shown by the CAST study for flecainide and encainide in adults with coronary heart disease [40]. However, pro-arrhythmia was also seen in 7–8 percent of children treated with these drugs [41]. Therefore, the risk of pro-arrhythmia should be considered, especially in patients with an impaired ventricular function. Finally, the cardiac depressant effect of many anti-arrhythmic drugs has to be considered, especially after a Fontan operation, after physiologic correction of transposition of the great arteries and in patients with inoperable heart disease.

The conversion and prevention of atrial flutter with drugs in this group of patients is comparable to the treatment used in adults. Digitalis should nearly always be combined with, or replaced by, verapamil or a beta blocker to control AV conduction, and even then 1:1 conduction may occur. Therefore, termination of atrial flutter is the aim of the treatment. Type III drugs such as sotalol and amiodarone, type IA drugs such as quinidine and type IC drugs such as flecainide and propafenone are capable of terminating and preventing the recurrence of atrial flutter. Type IA and IC drugs should always be combined with a drug that slows AV conduction to prevent 1:1 conduction when the flutter rate is slowed by the IA and IC drugs.

DC Cardioversion and pacing

DC Cardioversion and endocardial or trans-esophageal overdrive pacing are good methods for acute termination of atrial flutter. However, in DC cardioversion back-up pacing is often necessary to prevent severe bradycardia or arrest. Electrical cardioversion is usually preferable to prolonged trials with drugs.

As mentioned earlier the main indication for pacemaker implantation in this group is the brady-tachy syndrome in patients who need drug treatment for tachycardia, as well as some cases of symptomatic bradycardia or congenital or surgical AV block. If AV conduction is normal, AAI pacing is preferable. Especially after a Fontan operation, but also after the physiologic correction of transposition, the contribution of AV synchrony in cardiac output is important. Moreover, Silka et al. [42] found that in patients with congenital heart disease, atrial pacing decreases the incidence of bradycardia-mediated tachycardia. Unfortunately the prevention of atrial flutter was less clear than of supraventricular tachycardia and ventricular tachycardia. If atrial flutter recurs despite pacing, AAI pacing is useless unless the pacemaker has automatic anti-tachycardia facilities. Many patients with the brady-tachy syndrome have an impaired heart rate response to exercise. AAI-R pacing is the preferred mode in these patients to improve their exercise capacity and to prevent tachycardia. Unfortunately the combination of rate-responsive and anti-tachycardia pacing is not yet available, but it could improve the management of these patients.

Pacemaker implantation in patients with congenital heart disease produces more problems than in adults with normal hearts. An often unexpected finding is moderate or severe stenosis of the superior vena cava in 10–20 percent of the patients after physiologic correction of transposition of the great arteries. Therefore, the superior vena cava should be visualized before implantation, e.g. by a digital subtraction angiogram. The right atrial appendage is often used for cannulation and belongs to the pulmonary venous atrium in patients after the Mustard operation. Therefore, use of an electrode with active fixation is usually required in the atrium. Moreover, the atrial wall contains scars and prosthetic material, which often interferes with the finding of a good sensing – and stimulation threshold. If ventricular pacing is indicated in patients after a Mustard or Senning operation, the ventricular lead has to be placed in the smooth anatomic left ventricle, making active fixation necessary (Figure 4). In patients after a Fontan operation, the ventricle can only be stimulated epicardially, and after a total cavopulmonary connection neither the atrium nor the ventricle can be stimulated endocardially. If there is any suspicion of conduction abnormalities or arrhythmias at the end of these types of operation, permanent epicardial leads should be placed to prevent a second thoracotomy. If these technical aspects are taken into account, pacing of people with (operated) congenital heart disease is quite feasible [43–46].

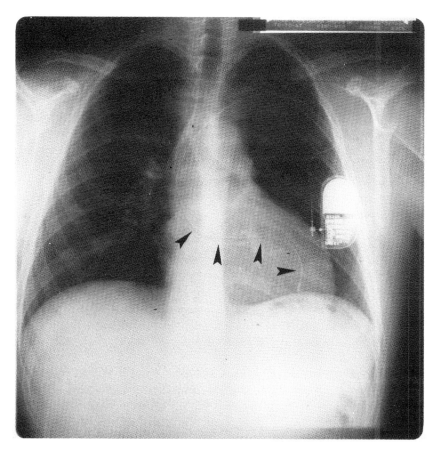

Figure 4. An endocardial pacemaker electrode in the anatomic left ventricle in a patient after a Mustard operation.

Surgery and ablation

The electrophysiologic mechanism of atrial flutter is complicated and has not yet been completely unravelled, but large reentrant loops and areas of conduction delay play a role. Guiraudon et al. [47] used cryo-ablation of the area of slow conduction near the coronary sinus, guided by endocardial mapping. Two of the 3 patients with atrial flutter were treated successfully. Touboul and colleagues [48] performed catheter ablation of the area with fragmented potentials in the low posteroseptal atrium during sustained flutter. Treatment was a success in 5 of 8 patients. There is not yet experience with these techniques in people with congenital heart disease, but further development of these methods could well become important for the treatment of atrial flutter after cardiac surgery. Surgical or catheter ablation of the atrioventricular node can be a final form of treatment for uncontrollable atrial flutter. It is hoped that the above-mentioned more recent techniques will be capable of solving the problem of atrial flutter more elegantly in the future.

Conclusions

Supraventricular arrythmias in congenital heart disease are caused by altered hemodynamics and by surgical injury of the conduction system, especially the sinus node and the sinus node artery. The sinus node dysfunction combined with fibrosis and scarring of the atrial wall often results in a brady-tachy syndrome. The incidence of supraventricular arrhythmias is highest after physiologic correction of transposition of the great arteries and the Fontan operation, and increases with the length of follow-up. Patients with uncontrolled atrial flutter are at risk for sudden death. Therefore, treatment should be directed at termination and prevention of atrial flutter by cardioversion, anti-tachy pacing, drugs or ablation techniques. More recent surgical techniques such as the anatomic correction of transposition of the great arteries and the total cavopulmonary connection may reduce the incidence of postoperative supraventricular arrhythmias.

References

1. Bharati S, Lev M, Kirklin JW. Cardiac surgery and the conduction system. New York : John Wiley and Sons, Inc, 1983:2–6.
2. Smith A, Arnold R, Wilkinson JL, Hamilton DI, McKay R, Anderson RH. An anatomical study of the patterns of the coronary arteries and sinus nodal artery in complete transposition. Int J Cardiol 1986;12:295–304.
3. Rossi MB, Ho SY, Anderson RH, Rossi Filho RI, Lincoln C. Coronary arteries in complete transposition: The significance of the sinus node artery. Ann Thorac Surg 1986;42:573–7.
4. Battistessa SA, Ho SY, Anderson RH, Smith A, Deverall PB. The arterial supply to the right atrium and the sinus node in classic tricuspid atresia. J Thorac Cardiovasc Surg 1988;96:816–22.

5. Boyden PA, Tilley LP, Pham TD, Liu SK, Fenoglio JJ, Wit AL. Effects of left atrial enlargement on atrial transmembrane potentials and structure in dogs with mitral valve fibrosis. Am J Cardiol 1982;49:1896–1908.

6. Wittig JH, de Leval MR, Stark J, Castaneda A. Intraoperative mapping of atrial activation before, during, and after the Mustard operation. J Thorac Cardiovasc Surg 1977;73:1–13.

7. Anderson RH, Ho SY, Becker AE. The surgical anatomy of the conduction tissues. Thorax 1983;38:408–20.

8. Clark EB, Kugler JD. Preoperative secundum atrial septal defect with coexisting sinus node and atrioventricular node dysfunction. Circulation 1982;65:976–80.

9. Ruschhaupt DG, Khoury L. Thilenius OG, Replogle RL, Arcilla RA. Electrophysiologic abnormalities of children with ostium secundum atrial septal defect. Am J Cardiol 1984;53:1643–7.

10. Vetter VL, Tanner CS, Horowitz LN. Electrophysiologic consequences of the Mustard repair of d-transposition of the great arteries. J Am Coll Cardiol 1987;6:1265–73.

11. Kurer CC, Tanner CS, Vetter VL. Electrophysiologic consequences of Fontan repair. Am J Cardiol 1988;62:510 (abstr).

12. Lucet V, Batisse A, Ngoc DD, et al. Troubles du rythme apres corrections atriales des transpositions des gros vaisseaus. Arch Mal Coeur 1986;79:640–7.

13. Vetter VL, Tanner CS, Horowitz LN. Inducible atrial flutter after the Mustard repair of complete transposition of the great arteries. Am J Cardiol 1988;61:428–35.

14. Bink-Boelkens MThE, Velvis H, Homan van der Heide JJ, Eygelaar A, Hardjowijono R. Dysrhythmias after atrial surgery in children. Am Heart J 1983;106:125–30.

15. Hamilton WT, Haffajee CI, Dalen JE, et al. Atrial septal defect secundum: Clinical profile and physiological correlates in children and adults. Cardiovasc Clin 1979;10:267.

16. Rosketh R. Congenital heart disease in middle-aged adults. Acta Med Scand 1968;183:131.

17. Brandenburg RO, Holmes DR, Brandenburg RO, McGoon DC. Clinical follow-up study of paroxysmal supraventricular tachyarrhythmias after operative repair of a secundum type atrial septal defect in adults. Am J Cardiol 1983;51:273–6.

18. Bink-Boelkens MThE, Meuzelaar KJ, Eygelaar A. Arrhythmias after repair of secundum atrial septal defect: The influence of surgical modification. Am Heart J 1988;115:629–33.

19. Friedman RA. Unoperated congenital and acquired heart disease. In: Gillette PC, Garson Jr A, editors. Pediatric arrhythmias, electrophysiology and pacing. Philadelphia: WB Saunders Comp, 1990;655–67.

20. Dubrow I, Fisher E, Thanopoulos B, et al. Electrophysiologic effects of cyanosis on sinus node and atrium in children. Circulation 1977;56, 57:suppl III–172.

21. Gillette PC, Shannon C, Garson A Jr, et al. Pacemaker treatment of sick sinus syndrome in children J Am Coll Cardiol 1983;1:1325–9.

22. Bharati S, Lev M. Sudden death long after repair of atrial septal defect: A study of four cases. Circulation 1986;74:II–121 (abstr).

23. Flinn CF, Wolff GS, Dick MD, et al. Cardiac rhythm after the Mustard operation for complete transposition of the great arteries. N Eng J Med 1984;310:1635–8.

24. Hayes CJ, Gersony WM. Arrhythmias after the Mustard operation for transposition of the great arteries: A long-term study. Ped Cardiol 1986;7:133–7.

25. Bogaards M, Dick M, Robinson B, et al. Late arrhythmias and outcome in patients after the Mustard operation for transposition of the great arteries: Update of 1981 Pediatric electrophysiology group collaborative study. Circulation 1990;82:III–223 (abstr.).

26. Gewillig M, Cullen S, Mertens B, Lesaffre E, Deanfield J. Risk factors for death after Mustard operation for simple transposition of the great arteries. Circulation 1990;82:III–77 (abstr).

27. Edwards WD, Edwards JE. Pathology of the sinus node in d-transposition following the Mustard operation. J Thorac Cardiovasc Surg 1978;75:213–8.

28. Bink-Boelkens MThE, Bergstra A, Cromme-Dijkuis AH, Eygelaar A, Landsman MLJ, Mooyaart EL. The asymptomatic child a long time after the Mustard operation for transposition of the great arteries. Ann Thorac Surg 1989;47:45–50.

29. Wernovksy G, Jonas RA, Mayer JE, Hanley FL, Castaneda AR. Results of the arterial switch operation in neonates. Circulation 1990;82:III–195 (abstr).

30. Vetter VL, Tanner CS. Electrophysiologic consequences of the arterial switch repair of d-transposition of the great arteries. J Am Coll Cardiol 1988;12:229–37.

31. Martin RP, Radley-Smith R, Yacoub MH. Arrhythmias before and after anatomic correction of transposition of the great arteries. J Am Coll Cardiol 1987;10:200–4.

32. Villafane J, White S, Elbl F, Rees A, Solinger R. An electrocardiographic midterm follow-up study after anatomic repair of transposition of the great arteries. Am J Cardiol 1990;66:350–4.

33. Weber HS, Hellenbrand WE, Kleinman CS, Perlmutter RA, Rosenfeld LE. Predictors of rhythm disturbances and subsequent morbidity after the Fontan operation. Am J Cardiol 1989;64:762–7.

34. Chen S, Nouri S, Pennington DG. Dysrhythmias after the modified Fontan operation. Ped Cardiol 1988;9:215–9.

35. Porter CJ, Battiste CE, Humes RA, et al. Risk factors for supraventricular tachyarrhythmias after Fontan procedure for tricuspid atresia. Am Heart J 1986;112:645 (abstr).

36. Gewillig M, Lundstrom U, Deanfield JE. Determinants and outcome of early and late arrhythmia after Fontan operation. J Am Coll Cardiol 1989;13:170A (abstr).

37. de Leval MR, Kilner P, Gewillig M, Bull C. Total cavopulmonary connection: A logical alternative to atriopulmonary connection for complex Fontan operations. J Thorac Cardiovasc Surg 1988;96:682–95.

38. Balaji S, Gewillig M, de Leval MR, Deanfield JE. Are postoperative arrhythmias after Fontan operation preventable by the total cavo-pulmonary connection? Circulation 1990;82:III–76 (abstr).

39. Garson A Jr, Bink-Boelkens M, Hesslein PS, et al. Atrial flutter in the young: A collaborative study of 380 cases. J Am Coll Cardiol 1985;6:871–8.

40. Cardiac Arrhythmia Suppression Trial Preliminary report: effect of encainide and flecainide on mortality in a randomized trial of arrhythmia suppression after myocardial infarction. N Eng J Med 1989;321:406–12.

41. Fish FA, Gillette PC, Benson DW. Incidence of death, cardiac arrest and proarrhythmia in young patients receiving flecainide or encainide. Circulation 1989;80:II–387 (abstr).

42. Silka MJ, Manwill JR, Kron J, McAnulty JH. Bradycadia-mediated tachyarrhythmias in congenital heart disease and responses to chronic pacing at physiologic rates. Am J Cardiol 1990;65:488–93.

43. Gillette PC, Wampler DG, Shannon C, Ott D. Use of atrial pacing in a young population. Pace 1985;8:94–100.

44. Case CL, Gillette PC, Zeigler V, Sade RM. Problems with permanent atrial pacing in the Fontan patient. Pace 1989;12:92–6.

45. Westerman GR, van Devanter SH. Surgical management of difficult pacing problems in patients with congenital heart disease. J Cardiac Surg 1987;2:351–60.

46. Taliercio CP, Vlietsra RE, McGoon MD, Porter CJ, Osborn MJ, Danielson GK. Permanent cardiac pacing after the Fontan procedure. J Thorac Cardiovasc Surg 1985;90:414–9.

47. Guiraudon GM, Klein GJ, Sharma AD, Yee R. Surgical alternatives for supraventricular tachycardias. Am J Cardiol 1989;64:92J–6J.

48. Touboul P, Saoudi N, Atallah G, Kirkorian G. Electrophysiologic basis of catheter ablation in atrial flutter. Am J Cardiol 1989;64:79J–82J.

11. Ventricular arrhythmias after repair of congenital heart disease: who needs treatment?

ARTHUR GARSON JR.

Introduction

Sudden death occurs in patients after repair of congenital heart disease. In those with tetralogy of Fallot, or a similar lesion, ventricular tachycardia has been hypothesized as the major arrhythmic mechanism for sudden death. It would be desirable to identify individuals at risk for sudden death, to determine which arrhythmia would be likely to cause sudden death, and to treat those individuals with an appropriate anti-arrhythmic to prevent sudden death. For the last 10 years, physicians have been treating patients with antiarrhythmic drugs, based on a number of criteria, the most common of which is the presence of premature ventricular contractions [1]. The practice has recently been called into question by the CAST trial. It is the purpose of this paper to review the evidence that repair causes ventricular arrhythmias, that ventricular arrhythmias cause sudden death and that ventricular arrhythmias should be treated prophylactically.

Repair causes ventricular arrhythmias

Since the majority of work has been done on postoperative tetralogy of Fallot, this analysis will confine itself to tetralogy of Fallot, recognizing that in most series, the more complex lesions (e.g. truncus arteriosus, double outlet right ventricle) have a higher mortality and the less complex lesions (e.g. VSD) have lower mortality. Since 1972, 39 studies have been published in the English language literature on 4,627 patients after repair of tetralogy of Fallot. Those comprising the largest number of patients are referenced [3–10]. In these studies, 8 percent of patients had premature ventricular contractions on routine electrocardiogram (range 1–33 percent), 18 percent on exercise test (range 13–45 percent), 46 percent on Holter (range 2–77 percent), and 17 percent had

John Hess and George R. Sutherland (eds.), Congenital Heart Disease in Adolescents and Adults, 147–154.

ventricular tachycardia induced at electrophysiology study (14–34 percent). The mean age at surgery was 7.3 years (range 1–13); the average age at followup was 16.7 years; this was 8.7 years after surgery. Sudden death occurred in 1.8 percent (range 0–5.5 percent). A number of factors were associated with the presence of ventricular arrhythmias: older age at surgery in 10/11 studies (91 percent), longer duration of followup (71 percent); however, when age and followup were analyzed together, in two studies it was found that the followup duration was the more significant factor rather than the age at surgery. Other factors included multiple repairs in 80 percent of studies, high right ventricular systolic pressure in 60 percent, high right ventricular end-diastolic pressure in 63 percent, reduced left ventricular function in 67 percent. Therefore, it appears that ventricular arrhythmias are present after surgery and that a number of factors are associated with these arrhythmias that might lead to sudden death.

However, Sullivan et al., in 1987 [11], challenged the concept that the arrhythmias develop postoperatively. They found that there were arrhythmias present before surgery. Then examined two groups of patients. In the first, the age was less than 7 years and none of these patients had ventricular arrhythmias on their Holter before surgery; 18 patients were over 13 years of age and 8/18 had premature ventricular contractions on their Holter before surgery. Four lines of evidence can be brought to bear to establish that ventricular arrhythmias are caused by the operation. Tamer et al. [12] demonstrated that 17 percent of postoperative patients had ventricular arrhythmias on routine electrocardiogram. The mean age of these patients was 8 years. Therefore, if we assume by Sullivan's data [11] that there were no preoperative ventricular arrhythmias in children less than 8 and since half of Tamer's patients were less than 8 with ventricular arrhythmias, we can assume that the surgery caused the arrhythmias in Tamer's patients [12]. Zimmerman [13] did a comparative study of late potentials and found that there were no late potentials before surgery, but late potentials developed after surgery. A third piece of evidence concerns the observations made Horowitz [14], Kugler [15] and Dunnigan [16] that a second repair increases the incidence of ventricular arrhythmias independent of age. Finally, when intracardiac electrophysiology studies are performed on postoperative tetralogy patients, the induced ventricular tachycardia is mapped to areas adjacent to surgical scar (Horowitz et al. [14], Kugler et al. [15], Swerdlow et al. [17]). If surgery did not cause ventricular arrhythmias, the ventricular tachycardia would map to a number of sites throughout the ventricle. Since the arrhythmias map adjacent to scar, it is likely that the scar was somehow related to the ventricular arrhythmias. Finally, on an experimental level, Erickson has demonstrated in a postoperative tetralogy dog model that ventricular arrhythmias develop in animals after cardiopulmonary bypass and repair of simulated tetralogy of Fallot, whereas no ventricular arrhythmias are present before surgery (unpublished data). In this animal model, sudden death has occurred in one animal after repair with premature ventricular contractions, increased right ventricular systolic pressure and pulmonary insufficiency. Therefore, while it may be possible that certain teenage patients develop premature ventricular contractions before repair of tetralogy of Fallot, the majority of patients who have ventricular arrhythmias do so after repair and these arrhythmias are related to the repair.

It has recently been hypothesized that as long as surgery is performed at a young age, ventricular arrhythmias may not develop. Walsh et al. [18] studied a group of patients all operted upon under 18 months of age and found that only 2 percent had ventricular arrhythmias on Holter. The followup at the time of the Holter was five years. However, Chandar [19] and Benito [20] have demonstrated in larger series of patients that ventricular arrhythmias were more closely associated with followup rather than age at surgery. Sullivan [11] demonstrated that ventricular arrhythmias increase with puberty. Denfield et al. [21] have provided an experimental basis for this observation. A right ventriculotomy was performed in puppies of three different ages: newborn, young puppies 2 months of age and adult dogs. They found that in the newborn and young puppies, the scar length grew by approximately 200 percent, wheres in the adults dogs, the scar shrank by 20 percent (p less than 0.05). These investigators speculated that a cricital mass of scar tissue provided the substrate for ventricular arrhythmias. On the basis of these studies, it appears that ventricular arrhythmias may develop even in those operated upon at a young age. We will have to await a long-term followup study until these young patients have undergone puberty before we will be able to assess these results in perspective.

Ventricular arrhythmias cause sudden death

Among the 4,627 patients reported, 57 (1.8 percent) died suddenly. Certain factors were found to be associated with sudden death (Table 1). As can be seen from the data, ventricular arrhythmias are statistically related to sudden

Table 1. Postoperative tetralogy of fallot factors associated with sudden death.

Symptoms	Sudden death N = 57 18%	Alive N = 4570 —	P
V Arr Routine ECG	61%	8%	0.001
Exercise test	50%	18%	0.001
Holter	93%	46%	0.001
EPS	38%	17%	0.01
RVSP	77%	20%	0.001
RVEDP	85%	20%	0.001
Abnormal Hem + V Arr on Holter	80%	8%	0.0001

death, as are abnormal hemodynamics. However, ventricular arrhythmias and abnormal hemodynamics are also found in patients who do not die suddenly. Statistically, the best single pedictor for sudden death is the combination of abnormal hemodynamics and ventricular arrhythmias on Holter (Lown grade II or more). Even using this combination as a risk factor, 80 percent of those with sudden death had the combination of abnormal hemodynamics with ventricular arrhythmias whereas only 8 percent of those who were alive had this combination (p less than 0.001). As can be seen from the Table, symptoms are a poor predictor. Only 18 percent of patients who later died suddenly had symptoms before their death. Additionally, Ewing [22] and Chandar [19] found that symptoms were present in a number of patients without ventricular arrhythmias and who did not later die suddenly. These symptoms are neither sensitive nor specific. Of note is the fact that inducible ventricular arrhythmias are not a risk factor for sudden death. In the recent study by Chandar et al. [19], 370 patients underwent intracardiac electrophysiology studies after repair of tetralogy of Fallot; five of these died suddenly and none had had induced ventricular tachycardia.

Clinical studies also support the concept that ventricular arrhythmias also cause sudden death. Deanfield [23] examined the hearts of five patients who died suddenly. He found that there was right ventricular fibrosis present and that the conduction systems were normal. Therefore since sudden death has been hypothesized to occur either because of AV block or ventricular tachycardia associated with fibrosis, it is likely that in these patients, since the conduction system was normal, their deaths were caused by ventricular tachycardia. A second line of evidence has demonstrated that if patients with known ventricular arrhythmias are treated, the incidence of sudden death decreases. Specifically, Dunnigan [16] and Swerdlow [17] have treated patients with symptoms or cardiac arrest due to documented ventricular tachycardia and when the ventricular arrhythmias were treated, the symptoms and cardiac arrests did not recur. Finally, while ventricular arrhythmias in this patient population are known to be a risk factor, it is also known that patients with abnormal hemodynamics are prone to develop atrial flutter [24]. It is, therefore, possible that atrial flutter caused some of these deaths. On the other hand, since the majority of treatment used for ventricular arrhythmias (phenytoin, mexiletin, propranolol) are not usually effective in atrial flutter, the conclusion could be reached that since the postoperative tetralogy patients become asymptomatic and have no further episodes of cardiac arrest on this type of treatment, then the initiating arrhythmia was not likely to be atrial flutter.

In the experimental laboratory, Dreyer et al. [25] have studied the plasma catecholamines in animals with different hemodynamics. Specifically, when animals with a pulmonary artery band and increased right ventricular systolic pressure underwent ventricular pacing at 240 per minute simulating ventricular tachycardia, the plasma norepinephrine levels approximately doubled whereas when the control animals underwent pacing at the same rate, there was not significant change in plasma norephiephrine. The change in plasma norepinephrine had a strong negative correlation with cardiac output during left ventricular pacing, i.e. as the cardiac output during pacing decreased in those animals with high right ventricular systolic and end-diastolic pressure, the plasma norepinephrine level increased. These authors speculated that in patients after repair of tetralogy of Fallot, if ventricular tachycardia develops on an electrophysiologic basis, the rapid rate results in a fall in cardiac output, an increase in plasma norepinephrine, thus causing a decrease in the ventricular fibrillation threshold, eventually allowing for the deterioration of ventricular tachycardia into ventricular fibrillation.

Ventricular arrhythmias should be treated prophylactically

An excellent way to analyze the risk-benefit ratio of a clinical problem is to use the mathematical method of decision analysis. The decision tree is shown in Figure 1. The statistics are all based on available data from the literature [3–10]. A high risk group can be identified that has greater than 30 PVCs per hour on Holter and abnormal hemodynamics (right ventricular systolic pressure greater than or equal to 60 mmHg or right ventricular end-diastolic pressure greater than or equal to 8 mmHg). Approximately 10 percent of all postoperative tetralogy patients are in this group [3–10]. If they are not treated, the mortality rate is 15 percent. If they are treated, approximately 20 percent will develop side effects from the treatment. Included in the number with side effects are the 5 percent of those with side effects who may die [26]. Therefore, comparing the different treatment strategies, with no treatment, 15 patients out of 1000 will die whereas only 1 out of 1000 will die with treatment.

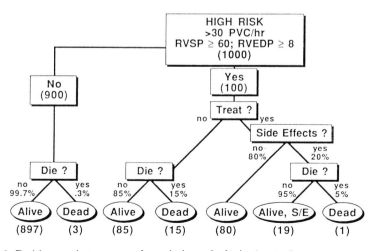

Figure 1. Decision tree in treatment of ventricular arrhythmias (see text).

On the other side, 90 percent of patients are not in the high risk group with ventricular arrhythmia and abnormal hemodynamics. None of these patients will be treated. Approximately 0.3 percent will die (3/1000). It can be seen that the overall death rate of untreated patients is 18/1000 (1.8 percent). This agrees with the figures in the literature [3–10]. Therefore, by this mathematical analysis, it can be seen that prophylactic treatment of ventricular arrhythmias of at least Lown grade II in the high risk subgroup of those with accompanying abnormal hemodynamics, is justified.

Current practice – texas children's hospital

There are not enough data presently available to answer the question of specifically which single patient requires treatment. Our current practice is based upon the risk-benefit ratio considering that we treat most of these patients with relatively 'benign' drugs with a low incidence of proarrhythmia (e.g. phenytoin, mexiletine, propranolol). Our general concept is to use both hemodynamics and presence of ventricular arrhythmias on Holter as a consideration for treatment. Intracardiac electrophysiology study is used only as an adjunct, since recent data have shown a low sensitivity and specificity for electrophysiologic testing in postoperative tetralogy patients [19]. We currently approach treatment in the following way: if symptoms are present regardless of the Holter findings or hemodynamics, electrophysiology study is done. The major reason for doing the electrophysiology study is to exclude other possible causes of syncope in a postoperative tetralogy patient (i.e. atrial flutter, AV block). If ventricular tachycardia is induced, repeat electrophysiology study is done with the patient on drugs to determine if the drug effectively eliminates the inducibility of ventricular tachycardia. Regardless of the electrophysiologic findings, if any more than 1000 PVCs per day or complex ventricular arrhythmias are present on the Holter, these are treated unless another cause for the syncope can be documented.

The remainder of the discussion concerns the asymptomatic patient. Patients with less than 1000 PVCs per day are not treated regardless of their hemodynamics. They do not undergo electrophysiology study. In those with Lown grade II–III on their Holter, if the hemodynamics are good, electrophysiology study is not performed and the patient is not treated. If ventricular arrhythmias of Lown grade II–III are present and the hemodynamics are bad, the patient undergoes electrophysiologic testing as a baseline for a drug study, but no decision is reached about treatment based upon the electrophysiology study. In these patients, the goal is to suppress inducibility of ventricular arrhythmias and to suppress ventricular arrhythmia on the Holter by Morganroth's criteria [27]. Finally, if the patient has Lown grade IV–V ventricular arrhythmia and good hemodynamics, then a diagnostic electrophysiologic study is performed. If there is inducible sustained monomorphic ventricular tachycardia, the patient then undergoes drug testing and drug election on the basis of suppression of indicibility. Attempts are also made to suppress PVCs on the Holter. If the patient has Lown grade IV–V ventricular arrhythmias and poor hemodynamics, then electrophysiology study is performed, but the study is performed for a baseline for treatment rather than for diagnosis.

Conclusions

Ventricular arrhythmias after repair of tetralogy of Fallot result in sudden death. It is clear that they should be suppressed in high risk patients. A major problem is the identification of the high risk patient. Unfortunately, we cannot use the data from adults with coronary artery disease to determine which patient should be treated after repair of congenital heart disease. The substrate is different and the hemodynamics are different. Similarly, while the CAST trial provides the basis for reluctance in the prophylactic treatment of ventricular arrhythmias, it does not necessarily apply to patients who have had repair of tetralogy of Fallot. While the conclusion from the CAST study were clear, the far ranging implications may be less than originally thought. For example, it may simply be that encainide and flecainide were arrhythmogenic in the particular subpopulation of patient in which they were used in the CAST study. These data should not be taken to imply that the 'PVC hypothesis' is incorrect, but perhaps that less arrhythmogenic drugs need to be found.

A 1.8 percent mortality rate over 8.4 years is a relatively low number; therefore, in order to demonstrate a positive effect of a drug on the prevention of sudden death, an extremely large (much larger than CAST) multicenter study will need to be conducted with a double blind placebo controlled design. Since there is uncertainty as to who needs to be treated, the placebo arm is important. However, until such a study is underway, personal preferences will prevail. I would rather explain to a parent of a child who had died on medication that we were trying to save his life rather than to explain to a parent of the untreated patient that we did not try. 'A low incidence of sudden death is only a statistic as long as it is not your child'.

References

1. Garson A, Randall DG, McVey P, et al. Prevention of sudden death after repair of tetralogy of Fallot: Treatment of ventricular arrhythmias. J Am Coll Cardiol 1985;6:221–7.
2. Fish FA, Gillette PC, Benson DW. Incidence of death, cardiac arrest and proarrhythmia in young patients receiving flecainide or encainide. Circulation 1989;80:II–387.
3. Wolff GS, Rowland TW, Ellison RC. Surgically induced right bundle branch block with left anterior hemiblock: An ominous sign in postoperative tetralogy of Fallot. Circulation 1972;46:587–94.
4. James FW, Kaplan S, Chou T. Unexpected cardiac arrest in patients after surgical correction of tetralogy of Fallot. Circulation 1975;52:691–5.

5. Quattlebaum TG, Varghese J, Neill CA. Sudden death among postoperative patients with tetralogy of Fallot. A follow-up study of 243 patients for an average of 12 years. Circulation 1976;54:289–93.

6. Garson A, Nihill MR, McNamara DG, Cooley DA. Status of the adult and adolescent following repair of tetralogy of Fallot. Circulation 1979;59:1232–40.

7. Fuster V, McGoon DC, Kirklin JW. Long-term evaluation (12–22 years) of open heart surgery for tetralogy of Fallot. Am J Cardiol 1980;46:635–42.

8. Deanfield JE, McKenna WJ, Hallidie-Smith KA. Detection of late arrhythmia and conduction distrubance after correction of tetralogy of Fallot. Br Heart J 1980;44:248–53.

9. Katz NM, Blackstone EH, Kirklin JW. Late survival and symptoms after repair of tetralogy of Fallot. Circulation 1982;65:403–10.

10. Miyamura H, Kanazawa H, Matsukawa T. Long-term postoperative status of tetralogy of Fallot. Jpn Circ J 1986;50:855–8.

11. Vaksmann G, Fournier A, Davignon A. Incidence and prognosis of arrhythmias in post-operative tetralogy of Fallot: Long-term follow-up study. Circulation 1988;80:II–597.

12. Sullivan ID, Presbitero P, Deanfield JE. Is ventricular arrhythmia in repaired tetralogy of Fallot an effect of operation or a consequence of the course of the disease? Br Heart J 1987;58:40–4.

13. Tamer D, Wolff GS, Gelband H. Hemodynamics and intracardiac conduction after operative repair of tetralogy of Fallot. Am J Cardiol 1983;51:552–6.

14. Zimmermann M, Friedli B, Oberhansli I. Frequency of ventricular late potentials and factioned right ventricular electrograms after operative repair of tetralogy of Fallot. Am J Cardiol 1987;59:448–53.

15. Horowitz LN, Vetter VL, Harken AH, Josephson ME. Electrophysiologic characteristics of sustained ventricular tachycardia occurring after repair of tetralogy of Fallot. Am J Cardiol 1980;46:446–52.

16. Kugler JD, Pinsky WW, Fleming WH. Sustained ventricular tachycardia after repair of tetralogy of Fallot: New electrophysiologic findings. Am J Cardiol 1983;51:1137–43.

17. Dunnigan A, Benditt DL, Benson DW. Life threatening ventricular tachycardias in late survivors of surgically corrected tetralogy of Fallot. Br Heart H 1984;52:198–206.

18. Swerdlow CD, Oyer PE, Pitlcik PT. Septal origin of sustained ventricular tachycardia in a patient with right ventricular outflow tract obstruction after correction of tetralogy of Fallot. PACE 1986;9:585–8.

19. Walsh EP, Keane JF, Hougen TJ. Late results in patients with tetralogy of Fallot repaired during infancy. Circulation 1988;77:1062–7.

20. Chandar JS, Wolff GS, Garson A. Ventricular arrhythmias in postoperative tetralogy of Fallot. Am J. Cardiol 1990;65:655–61.

21. Deal BJ, Scagliotti D, Levitsky J. Electrophysiologic drug testing in symptomatic ventricular arrhythmias after repair of tetralogy of Fallot. Am J Cardiol 1987;59:1380–5.

22. Denfield SW, Kearney DL, Michael L, Gittenberger-de Groot A, Garson A. Growth in cardiac surgical scars with age: A canine model. J Am Coll Cardiol 1990;15:176A.

23. Ewing L, Gillette PC. Only 8% of postoperative tetralogy patients have inducible dysrhythmias. J. Am Coll Cardiol 1987;9:36A.

24. Deanfield JE, Anderson RH, Hallidie-Smith KA. Late sudden death after repair of tetralogy of Fallot: a clinicopathologic study. Circulation 1983;67:626–31.

25. Garson A, Bink-Boelkens, Hesslein PS, Hordoff AJ, Keane JF, Neches WH, Porter CJ. Atrial flutter in the young: a collaborative study of 380 cases. J Am Coll Cardiol 1985;6:871–8.

26. Dreyer WJ, Paridon SM, Varughese A, Fisher DJ, Garson A. Serum norepinephrine elevation in dogs with high right ventricular pressure during simulated ventricular tachycardia. Am J Cardiol 1987;60(1):639.

27. Garson A, Gillette PC. Treatment of chronic ventricular dysrhythmias in the young. PACE 1981;4:658–69.

28. Morganroth J, Michelson EL, Horowitz LN. Limitations of routine long-term electrocardiographic monitoring to assess ventricular ectopic frequency. Circulation 1978;58:408–13.

12. Infective endocarditis: treatment and prophylaxis

JACOB DANKERT

Introduction

In infective endocarditis (IE) there is infection of the endocardium generally a heart valve, but infection may also occur on septal defects, the mural endocardium, a prosthetic heart valve, intracardiac patches, surgically constructed intracardiac shunts or in the tissues into which prostheses are sewn. IE of native endocardium which may be previously normal or abnormal due to congenital malformation of the heart or acquired disease, is referred to as native endocarditis. Prosthetic endocarditis (PE) refers to infection associated with the intracardiac prosthesis.

The frequency of IE difficult to ascertain because of the varying criteria used, ranges from 0.16 to 5.4 per 1000 hospital admissions, with a mean of approximately one case/1000 hospital admissions [1]. In a Dutch University Hospital (Groningen) IE, using strict case definitions [2], was diagnosed in 1.39 patients per 1000 hospital admissions in a ten years' survey from 1980 through 1989 (Dankert and Hess, unpublished). The estimated frequency for pediatric patients was 0.7 per 1000 admissions.

Previously, IE was most prevalent in patients younger than 35 years. Now it appears to become a disease of the middle-aged and the elderly [2]. The major exception to the aging population with IE will be intravenous drug abusers [3].

Almost any cardiac abnormality causing turbulence of the blood flow may predispose to IE. But in recent series 15 percent [2] to 43 percent [4] of the patients with IE had a normal or apparently normal heart before the onset of the disease. Left-sided IE is much more common than right-sided. The incidence of right-sided endocarditis, ranging from 2 to 15 percent of the cases [5], has increased with the increase of intravenous drug abuse [3] and the use of intravenous catheters [6]. The use of various intravascular devices is associated with a new form of IE namely hospital-acquired or nosocomial IE.

John Hess and George R. Sutherland (eds.), Congenital Heart Disease in Adolescents and Adults, 155–170.
© *1992 Kluwer Academic Publishers. Printed in the Netherlands.*

In a recent study nosocomial endocarditis accounted for 14 percent of cases [7]. In our series 38 (22%) of 175 patients with IE developed the disease secondary to various procedures in the hospital.

PE constitutes 12 to 33 percent of cases of IE [3]. In our series 63 (36%) of 175 patients with IE had early-onset or late-onset PE. Early-onset PE is commonly defined as infection occurring within 60 days of surgery, subsequent infection is late-onset. However, clinical manifestations of *Staphylococcus epidermidis* endocarditis related to heart surgery may become apparent one year after surgery.

The mortality of IE is still high. However, the outcome of the various forms of IE differs considerably. Overall mortality in native IE ranges from approximately 10 to 20 percent. There is differential mortality according to the nature of the infecting organism, the age of the patient and duration of symptoms prior to treatment [3]. The mortality of *Staphylococcus aureus* endocarditis is 30 to 40 percent, in enterococcal endocarditis 15 to 30 percent and in viridans streptococcal endocarditis 6 to 10 percent. Of the elederly over age 60, 30 to 40 percent of the patients with IE die because of the disease, whilst under age 40 the mortality of patients with IE is 8 to 12 percent [8]. Overall mortality of PE was as high as 50 to 70 percent. Mortality for early-onset PE has fallen from around 70 percent in the 1970s and early 1980s to about 30 percent in the last decade and for late-onset PE from 45 percent to 25 percent. This reduction in mortality has been ascribed to more widely practised surgical intervention in active PE. The outcome for patients with hospital-acquired endocarditis is still poor [2, 7]. The overall mortality is approximately 40 percent and more than 50 percent among cases over age 60.

The purpose of this report is to review the initial antimicrobial therapy of IE in relation to etiology and diagnostic features. Aspects of resistance against antibiotics recommended for specific therapy will be considered in the light of the resulting therapeutic dilemmas for IE. Briefly prevention of IE will be discussed, as well as monitoring the effect and duration of treatment.

Etiology of infective endocarditis

Native endocarditis

Gram-positive cocci like streptococci and staphylococci account for about 60 to 80 percent and 20 to 40 percent, respectively of culture-positive cases (Table 1). Streptococci are a heterogeneous group of microorganisms: viridans streptococci, roup D streptococci and beta-hemolytic streptococci. Viridans streptococci residing in the oral cavity, but some species are also found among the gut flora, is speciated into six to ten species. Identifying a viridans streptocococcal isolate is more than a taxonomic exercise. Certain species produce excessive amounts of exopolysaccharides. This leads to a decrease in the efficacy of penicillin on streptococcal endocarditis [9].

Table 1. Proportion (%) of predominant microorganisms causing native endocarditis. Data from literature and a prospective 10 years' survey at the University Hospital Groningen (UHG).

Microorganism	From literature [5]	UHG 1980–1989 (n = 112)
Viridans streptococci	40–50	51
Streptococcus sanguis	25–35	37
Streptococcus mitior	20–35	37
Streptococcus mitis	15–20	18
Streptococcus mutans	10–15	2
Streptococcus milleri	5–10	5
Streptococcus salivarius	1–5	2
Group D strepcococci	15–25	10
Enterococcus faecalis	30–45	55
Enterococcus faecium	5–10	0
Enterococcus durans	1–2	0
Streptococcus bovis	35–40	45
Streptococcus equinus	1–2	0
Other streptococci	2–5	5
Staphylococci	20–35	17
Coagulase-negative staphylococci	1–5	6
Other	5–10	5
Culture-negative	1–5	6

Streptococcus milleri has a greater capacity to give rise to metastatic infection than the other species. In addition, we assessed that *Streptococcus sanguis* (biotype I) and the majority of *Streptococcus mitior* isolates causing endocarditis exhibit tolerance to penicillin (see section specific treatment). In our series *S. sanguis* and *S. mitior* were responsible for 74 percent of the viridans streptococcal endocarditis cases, in adults as well as in pediatric cases (Table 1).

Group D enterococci, residing mainly in the gut, but also in the oral cavity, are also common in the etiology of native endocarditis (Table 1). In our series these bacteria predominantly *Enterococcus faecalis* and *Streptococcus bovis*, accounted for 10 percent of cases and caused 15 percent of the streptococcal cases (Table 1).

Speciation of group D enterococci is also relevant, because *S. bovis* endocarditis frequently is associated with pathological conditions of the gut, including carcinoma of the gut and because *Enterococcus* spp are resistant to many antibiotics whilst *S. bovis* is uniformly susceptible to penicillin.

Other streptococci causing 2 to 5 percent of native endocarditis cases, belong to beta-hemolytic streptococci, mainly groups B or G. These streptococci have a high potential for rapid valve destruction and myocardial abscess formation.

Staphylococci, mainly residing on the skin and the nasopharynx includes the coagulase-positive *S. aureus* and the coagulase-negative staphylococci, of which *Staphylococcus epidermidis* commonly is associated with PE and infrequently with native endocarditis. In contrast, *S. aureus* is the second cause of native endocarditis (Table 1). In intravenous drug addicts *S. aureus* is the single most common cause of native endocarditis and has a predilection for the right side of the heart, especially the tricuspid valve. *S. aureus* infects often a previously normal heart.

Native endocarditis, like other forms of IE can be caused by virtually any microorganism. Therefore, the etiology shows an array of bacterial species and various fungi. In our series *Haemophilus* spp were most often encountered among the various isolates other than streptococci and staphylococci.

Culture-negative endocarditis representing 1 to 5 percent of cases with native endocarditis refers to those patients from whom blood cultures remain negative. This may be attributable to improper culture techniques, but most frequently culture-negative endocarditis is associated with antibiotic therapy prior to the collection of blood samples for culturing. In our series a rather high proportion of endocarditis cases had blood cultures without growth (Table 1). Of these 11 cases, six had prior antibiotics, two developed elevated antibody titres against *Coxiella burnetti* (Q fever) and one had raised antibody titres against *Chlamydia psittaci*, which declined three months after appropriate antimicrobial treatment.

Endocarditis associated with intravenous drug abuse

Native endocarditis in intravenous drug users is caused by *S. aureus* in more than half of the cases. Streptococci (viridans streptococci and enterococci) are recovered from about 20 percent. In contrast to endocarditis due to *S. aureus*, streptococcal endocarditis is mainly located in the left side of the heart. Aerobic Gram-negative bacilli and yeasts (fungi) relatively rare causes of IE in general, are relatively frequently isolated from drug addicts with endocarditis. In our series one patient was an intravenous drug abuser.

Hospital-acquired endocarditis

Nosocomial or hospital-acquired endocarditis develops in patients with a previously normal heart, or a cardiac abnormality, or a cardiac prosthesis [2, 7]. Predominantly staphylococci, *S. aureus* as well as *S. epidermidis* are recovered. In our series mainly *S. epidermidis* and *Enterococcus faecalis* were isolated from cases with nosocomial endocarditis. The majority of cases emerged in the intensive therapy unit secondary to the use of non-absorbable oral antibiotics, suppressing aerobic Gram-negative bacteria in the gut flora (selective decontamination). This prophylactic regimen results in heavy colonization with staphylococci and enterococci and apparently in conjunction with the use of intravascular devices, in endocardial infection.

Prosthetic endocarditis

The etiology of early-onset PE differs from that of late-onset PE. *S. epidermidis* is the single most common organism in early-onset PE, causing 30 to 74 percent of cases (Table 2). Streptococci are infrequently reported in review series [10]. In our series a high proportion (30%) of patients developed early-onset PE due to *Enterococcus* spp, secondary to the preventive use of non-absorbable antibiotics in the intensive therapy unit. In late-onset PE *Streptococci* spp predominate accounting for 31 to 44 percent of cases. In our series streptococci were more common than in review series [10]. Viridans streptococci caused 37 percent of late-onset PE, *S. bovis* 15 percent and *Enterococcus* spp 11 percent (Table 2). Staphylococci were less common than in review series [10]. The other microorganisms represents *Listeria mono-cytogenes*, *Micrococcus sedentarius* and *Haemophilus* spp. The patient with culture-negative PE had a Coxiella infection.

Table 2. Microbiology of prosthetic endocarditis. Data from literature and a prospective 10 years' survey at the University Hospital Groningen (UHG).

Microorganism	Early-onset (%)		Late-onset (%)	
	From literature [10]	UHG '80–'89 (n = 36)	From literature [10]	UHG '80–'89 (n = 27)
Staphylococcus epidermidis	30–74	48	4–31	11
Staphylococcus aureus	4–40	3	7–14	4
Gram-negative bacilli	2–20	3	2–23	4
Diphteroids (Coryne bacterium spp)	9–18	3	4–8	0
Streptococcus spp	⎧	6	⎧	37
Streptococcus bovis	⎨ 0–10	6	⎨ 31–44	15
Enterococcus spp	⎩	30	⎩	11
Fungi	2–14	0	0–8	0
Others	0–15	3	2–8	16
Culture-negative	0–2	0	0–1	4

Clinical features, diagnosis and initial treatment

Clinical presentation and diagnosis

IE is a disease that can only be diagnosed by examination of the endocardium or the tissue in which the cardiac prosthesis is sewn. Therefore in the clinical situation strict case definitions for the diagnosis should be applied [2].

The clinical presentation of the disease is non-specific. Most patients have some combination of fever and new or changing cardiac murmurs. In the elderly with IE poor febrile responses occur and new or changing cardiac murmurs are less frequently heard [8]. The paucity of clinical manifestations of the disease leads to a delay in the correct diagnosis [2, 8, 11]. Approximately in 30 percent of the cases with IE, the disease is not considered in the initial differential diagnosis [2] and in a rather high proportion the diagnosis is not entertained during hospital stay [8, 11]. In general, there is a considerable interval between the onset of signs of IE and the onset of adequate treatment, mainly due to physician delay [11]. Early diagnosis is of great prognostic relevance since the outcome of IE is influenced by the duration of symptoms before effective antibiotic treatment is started [2, 8, 11–13]. Echocardiography is recognized as the method of choice for the detection of valvular vegetations associated with IE. Transesophageal echocardiography superior over the transthoracic approach in the visualization of cardiac vegetations, improves the rate of detection of abscesses associated with endocarditis [14].

Bacteriological diagnosis

Bacteriological diagnosis of IE is based upon the continuous discharge of the causative microorganism in low numbers from the vegetation at the endocardial surface, into the blood stream. The percentage of positive cultures may, however, be influenced by prior antimicrobial therapy, the microorganism causing the disease and microbiological technique. Most cases of IE have positive blood cultures, when no antibiotic treatment prior to blood culturing is given. The bacteriological diagnosis in most cases with IE is made with the first blood culture obtained. However, the clinical importance of certain isolates can be best assessed when microorganisms are recovered from a number of cultures, performed at 30 to 60 min intervals. The major determinant of the yield of blood cultures collected, is the volume of blood cultured [15].

Therefore, it is preferable to collect three separate blood samples of 20 to 30 ml each for culturing. It has been shown that 95 percent of the first two blood cultures collected from patients with culture-positive endocarditis revealed growth [16]. If the three cultures remain negative, succeeding samples will rarely become culture-positive. There is possibly one exception. In patients who received antibiotic treatment prior to blood culturing, repeated blood culturing may resolve the causative microorganism if antibiotic treatment is delayed. But this can only be done if there is a hemodynamically stable patient with an history of an indolent begin of the disease, with no signs of emboli.

Generally, there is no need to wait upon the results of blood culture before starting treatment, when the clinical diagnosis of IE is made. In case of culture-negative blood samples serologic testing is the mainstay of diagnosing IE due to *C. burnetti*, *Chlamydia* spp, *Mycoplasma* spp, *Brucella* spp and *Legionella* spp. Serologic tests for the diagnosis of fungal endocarditis may be helpful.

Measurement of teichoic acid antibodies and circulating immunocomplexes may help to differentiate *S. aureus* bacteremia from bacteremia associated with *S. aureus* endocarditis [17]. Approximately three to six percent of patients with *S. aureus* bacteremia have endocarditis or will develop endocarditis [13], frequently without previous cardiac murmurs or cardiac abnormality.

Initial treatment

The decision which antibiotics should be chosen for the initial treatment is dependent on the course of IE, the type of IE and the presence of events predisposing of IE. Generally, the course of IE is associated with the virulent properties of the infecting microorganism. The type of IE and predisposing events may point to the presumptive etiology of the endocarditis.

General principles of antimicrobial treatment for IE are the following. Use antibiotics or combination of antibiotics with bactericidal effect, administer antibiotics parenterally, use established treatment regimens and do not compromise with respect to the duration of treatment. Community-acquired native endocarditis in patients with a history of heart disease and not addicted to intravenous drugs with an indolent begin and prolonged course, is predominantly due to viridans streptococci or group D streptococci. Initial treatment consists of high dose penicillin or amoxycillin plus gentamicin or netilmicin (Table 3). Native endocarditis in patients without a history of heart disease and not addicted to intravenous drugs with an abrupt begin and a fulminant illness with pyrexia is most likely due to *S. aureus*. Flucloxacillin in combination with gentamicin or netilmicin should be given to such patients (Table 3). If the infection is acquired in the hospital and methicillin resistant *S. aureus* (MRSA) is a possibility, vancomycin must be used.

Initial therapy for IE in intravenous drug abusers depends on the location of the infection in the heart. Right-sided IE is initially treated with flucloxacillin, whereas left-side IE is initially treated with flucloxacillin, amoxycillin plus gentamicin or netilmicin, because of the great variety of possible etiological microorganisms (Table 3).

Initial treatment of early-onset PE and hospital-acquired endocarditis consists of a combination of vancomycin, rifampicin plus gentamicin or netilmicin, irrespective the course (Table 3). Late-onset PE with an indolent begin and prolonged course is mainly due to viridans streptococci and *Enterococcus* spp. Initial treatment with a high dose of amoxycillin, vancomycin plus gentamicin or netilmicin is given (Table 3). If there is an abrupt begin and a fulminant course, patients are initially treated with flucloxacillin, rifampicin plus gentamicin [18] or with flucloxacillin, fusidic acid plus gentamicin or netilmicin [19] (Table 3).

Specific antibiotic treatment and antibiotic resistance yielding dilemmas in treatment of infective endocarditis

Antimicrobial therapy should be altered appropriately if necessary, when the causative microorganisms and results of susceptibility testing are known. Data for the specific treatment of IE are derived from the results of susceptibility tests in the laboratory, from experimental endocarditis studies in animals and from clinical studies. Recent excellent reviews correlating lessons from in vitro

Table 3. Initial treatment for infective endocarditis, after blood samples for culturing are collected and before results of culture and susceptibility tests are known.

Type of endocarditis	History of heart disease	Course and signs	Potential microorganism	Treatment (adult dose/24h)
Native	yes	indolent begin prolonged course	viridans streptococci Enterococcus spp S. bovis	penicillin 10–20 million U or amoxycillin 12 g plus gentamicin 240 mg or netilmicin 240 mg
Native	no	abrupt begin fulminant course	S. aureus	flucloxacillin 12 g plus gentamicin 240 mg or netilmicin 240 mg
Native right-sided in iv drug addicts	no	abrupt begin fulminant course pulmonary emboli	S. aureus	flucloxacillin 12 g
Native left-sided in iv drug addicts	yes	indolent begin prolonged course	Enterococcus spp viridans streptococci Ps. aeruginosa S. aureus	flucloxacillin 12 g plus amoxycillin 8 g plus gentamcin 240 mg or netilmicin 240 mg
Native left-sided in iv drug addicts	no	abrupt begin fulminant course	S. aureus	flucloxacillin 12 g
Prosthetic early-onset	—	indolent begin prolonged course as well as abrupt begin, fulminant course	S. epidermidis S. aureus	vancomycin 2 g plus rifampicin 900 mg plus gentamicin 240 mg or netilmicin 240 mg
Prosthetic late-onset	—	indolent begin prolonged course	viridans streptococci Enterococcus spp	amoxycillin 12 g plus vancomycin 2 g plus gentamicin 240 mg or netilmicin 240 mg
Prosthetic late-onset	—	abrupt begin fulminant course	S. aureus	flucloxacillin 12 g plus rifampicin 900 mg plus gentamicin 240 mg or netilmicin 240 mg

tests, the experimental studies and clinical studies are available [20, 21]. Therefore only recommended treatment regimens for the most common etiologic microorganisms will briefly be reviewed [18, 19].

Viridans streptococci

Viridans streptococci exhibit very low minimal inhibitory concentrations (MIC) for penicillin. Approximately only 20 percent of viridans streptococci are considered to be relatively resistant to penicillin on the basis of MICs, exceeding 0.1–0.2 mg/L, but below 1 mg/L. Concentrations of penicillin for which viridans streptococci are regarded as susceptible are a MIC of 0.1 mg/L in American reports [18] and a minimal bactericidal concentration (MBC) of 1 mg/L in British reports [19]. When treating IE it is widely accepted that it is necessary to kill the organism. Therefore the use of a MBC as a breakpoint to differentiate between fully susceptible and resistant viridans streptococci seems a reasonable approach. Concerning MBC values of viridans streptococci there is much controversy. A rather high proportion, ranging from 23 [22] to 80 percent [23] among viridans streptococcal isolates causing endocarditis have a high MBC for penicillin but a MIC of less than 0.1 mg/L. This discrepancy between MIC and MBC is called tolerance. We assessed that among viridans streptococci isolated from blood cultures of patients with endocarditis, 75 percent of the isolates were penicillin tolerant. According to British recommendations, treatment of patients with IE due to such strains is similar to patients with IE due to viridans streptococci with reduced susceptibility to penicillin [19]. Considering MICs these strains are susceptible and patients with IE due to tolerant viridants streptococcal strains can be treated with regimens as recommended recently for treatment of patients with IE due to penicillin susceptible viridans streptococci [18]. This may mean that treatment is done with penicillin along for 4 weeks, although it has been shown in experimental studies that treatment of IE due to tolerant strains with the combination of penicillin with an aminoglycoside, exerting synergistic killing in vitro, is superior to penicillin alone [21, 24, 25]. The recommendation [18] is in contrast to that for the treatment of IE due to viridans streptococci with MICs for penicillin between 0.1 and 0.5 mg/L. Treatment for IE caused by such strains has to be done with penicillin for four weeks plus gentamicin for the initial two weeks (Table 4), although through serum levels of penicillin achieved after high doses of intravenous penicillin exceeds MBCs of such non-tolerant strains.

Existing clinical data are inadequate basis for definitive recommendations regarding antibiotic therapy for IE due to either relatively penicillin resistant (MIC > 0.1 to < 0.5 mg/L) or penicillin tolerant (low MIC, high MBC) viridans streptococci [26]. We have treated patients with IE due to penicillin tolerant viridans streptococci with penicillin for at least 4 weeks with gentamicin or netilmicin for the first two weeks and achieved cure in all, except one who died due to congestive heart failure and emboli after surgery.

PE due to penicillin susceptible viridans streptococci should be treated with combination therapy of penicillin for at least six weeks and gentamicin or netilmicin for at least the first two weeks. Recommendations for treatment of PE due to penicillin (relatively) resistant and tolerant viridans streptococci are not available. We follow the recommendations as given for enterococcal endocarditis.

Enterococci and other group D streptococci

The MICs for penicillin of most enterococci are between 0.8 and 24 mg/L. A high proportion (50 percent) has MICs greater than 2 mg/L. All strains are intrinsically tolerant to penicillin and other cell-wall active antibiotics. The

Table 4. Suggested regimens for the treatment of infective endocarditis.

Type and cause of endocarditis	In USA		In Great Britain		
	Antibiotic	Duration (wks)	Microorganism	Antibiotic	Duration (wks)
NATIVE					
Viridans streptococci S. bovis with MICs ≤0.1 mg/L	penicillin or penicillin/ gentamicin or penicillin/ gentamicin	4 2/2 4/2	streptococci with MBCs ≤1 mg/L	penicillin/gentamicin (netilmicin) +oral amoxycillin	2/2 2
Viridans streptococci with MICs >0.1–0.5 mg/L	penicillin/ gentamicin	4/2	streptococci with MBCs >1 mg/L	penicillin/gentamicin (netilmicin)	4/2–4
Viridans streptocococci with MICs ⩾ 0.5 mg/L Enterococcus species	penicillin/ gentamicin or ampicillin (amoxycillin)/ gentamicin	4–6/4–6 4–6/4–6			
Staphylococcus species	flucloxa- cillin/ gentamicin	4–6/0.6	Staphylococcus species	flucloxacillin/ fusidic acid/ gentamicin (netilmicin)	4/4/2
PROSTHETIC					
Viridans streptococci	penicillin/ gentamicin	6/2	viridans streptocococci	penicillin/gentamicin	4–6/2–4
Staphylococcus species methicillin resistant	vancomycin/ gentamicin rifampicin	>6/2/>6	Staphylococcus species	flucloxacillin/ flusidic acid/gentamicin (netilmicin)	4–6/4–6/2
Methicillin susceptible	flucloxa– cillin/ rifampicin	>6/>6			

addition of gentamicin or netilmicin to penicillin, amoxycillin other beta-lactam antibiotics and vancomycin exerts a synergistic killing effect on enterococci. Therefore treatment of enterococcal endocarditis has focused on synergistic combinations.

The preferred treatment is penicillin plus gentamicin or amoxycillin plus gentamicin [18]. Treatment has to be continued for 4 to 6 weeks to achieve an overall cure rate of 75 percent. This recommended therapy has to be considered in the light of high-level resistance to gentamicin, eliminating the synergistic activity between penicillin and gentamicin (and other aminoglycosides as well). Patients with IE due to enterococci with this type of resistance and treated with the recommended therapy receive monotherapy with penicillin, yielding cure rates as low as 40 percent. High level gentamicin resistance can be easily transferred among strains. Another point of concern is the finding of enterococci producing beta-lactamase. These penicillin (and amoxycillin) resistant strains may be also resistant to gentamicin, leaving vancomycin as the only cell-wall active antibiotic with activity against enterococci. However, vancomycin resistant enterococci are also present [27]. Resistance to vancomycin is partly inducible and can be transferred among various bacterial species. Therefore it is not clear how long the recommended treatment regimens for enterococci will be useful.

S. bovis usually have low MICs for penicillin and treatment for endocarditis due to this microorganism is similar to treatment of endocarditis due to penicillin susceptible viridans streptococci.

PE due to enterococci is usually treated with high doses of amoxycillin for 6 weeks plus gentamicin for two to four weeks.

Staphylococcus aureus

S. aureus is rarely susceptible to penicillin. The recommended treatment for patients with native left-sided endocarditis due to S. aureus is flucloxacillin alone for 4 to 6 weeks or in combination with gentamicin (initial 2 weeks) according to American recommendations [18]. In Great Britain treatment with flucloxacillin plus fusidic acid or plus gentamicin or plus netilmicin is recommended [19]. Despite the synergistic action observed in vitro between flucloxacillin and gentamicin, the relevance of gentamicin in the treatment regimens is controversial. Combination thereapy has not achieved better cure rates than single therapy with flucloxacillin. In both cure rates ranged from 60 to 75 percent. Fusidic acid in combination with flucloxacillin was highly effective in treatment for IE due to S. aureus [28] but no comparative studies wih flucloxacillin alone are available. Right-sided endocarditis is most often treated with single therapy (flucloxacillin) for 4 weeks.

Problems encountered in the literature concerning S. aureus endocarditis are the increasing percentage of S. aureus strains resistant to flucloxacillin (so-called methicillin resistant, MRSA), the phenomenon of tolerance and the high rate of patients not responding to the instituted treatment. MRSA strains acquired a new gene that codes for the low-affinity penicillin binding protein 2a. Besides the problem of flucloxacillin resistance the strains show resistance to a large number of other antibiotics, including gentamicin. Treatment with vancomycin for 5 to 6 weeks is recommended for MRSA endocarditis. In the experimental endocarditis model it has been shown that amoxycillin clavulanate was more effective in the treatment of MRSA endocarditis than vancomycin [29]. Results of clinical trials comparing both antibiotics are not yet available.

Clinical trials have not shown that treatment of endocarditis due to tolerant *S. aureus* is impaired. However, in an experimental study cloxacillin was significantly less effective for treating endocarditis due to the tolerant *S. aureus* strain than the non-tolerant strains [30]. The high rate of patients not responding to the recommended treatment is caused by the extensive infection of the valve ring and the adjacent tissues frequently encountered in *S. aureus* endocarditis. Therefore the use of rifampicin has been suggested, because it exerts bactericidal activity against *S. aureus* in vitro, penetrates into abscesses and into leucocytes, killing phagocytosed viable bacteria. The drawback of rifampicin is that in vitro and in experimental studies its effect in combination with flucloxacillin, gentamicin or vancomycin is unpredictable. There may be an synergistic effect, an antagonistic effect or no effect. Therefore routine use of rifampicin is not recommended, but it may be used in patients not responding to the usual treatment.

PE due to *S. aureus* is treated with a combination of flucloxacillin for at least 6 weeks and gentamicin at least for the initial 2 weeks [18]. In the British recommendations fusidic acid is added to this combination. After gentamicin has been stopped, rifampicin may be added.

Coagulase-negative staphylococci

Endocarditis due to coagulase-negative staphylococci is predominantly associated with the presence of a cardiac prosthesis in the first year after valve insertion. A high proportion of these staphylococci is resistant to flucloxacillin. In addition, most PE due to those microorganisms are early-onset PE often due to multiply-resistant hospital-acquired strains. Treatment of PE due to coagulase-negative staphylococci is provided by the combination of vancomycin, rifampicin and gentamicin. Treatment with gentamicin is 2 to 4 weeks. Total duration of therapy is at least 6 weeks, but often longer. In approximately 20 to 50 percent of the strains resistance to gentamicin has been noted. When gentamicin has been stopped resistance to rifampicin may emerge. It may be that fusidic acid has a role in treatment of PE due to these bacteria, but clinical data of treatment regimens with fusidic acid are anecdotal.

Assessment of the response to therapy, duration and complications of treatment

Usually IE responds promptly to the antibiotics given. General malaise disappears and patients feel must better. However, the infection is still present and active in the heart. Fever can recur and intercurrent infection may occur complicating the clinical assessment of the response to treatment. To ascertain the effect of therapy the serum bactericidal test (SBT) is still widely used [31], despite there is little evidence that the results of this test can predict the adequacy of treatment. When SBT is done a peak serum bactericidal titer of at least 1:8 is mandatory in the treatment of IE.

Serial measurements of C-reactive protein (CRP) were found by us to be more useful than SBT to assess adequacy of therapy. In addition, rises in CRP concentrations pointed early to the onset of drug hypersensitivity and intercurrent infections. Such infections are those that one would expect with long-term high dose antibiotic therapy: infected venous access sites, catheter-associated bacteremia and fungemia, other fungal infections and pseudomembranous colitis due to *Clostridium difficile*. Pseudomembranous colitis as a complication of endocarditis treatment occurred in one of our 175 patients. As far as known no reports in the literature analyzing this complication as a consequence of antibiotic treatment of IE patients, are available.

Fever recurring after initial defervescence is rarely due to inadequate treatment, in contrast to fever persistence beyond the first 7 to 10 days of appropriate treatment [32]. Most patients with fever persistence have abscesses present in the valve ring and surrounding tissues [14, 32]. Usually surgical treatment is required in those patients [32]. Duration of treatment is difficult to predict. Many considerations affect the duration of treatment, such as which form of IE is present, which microorganism is responsible for the illness, which was the interval between the occurrence of the signs of IE and the start of therapy. In the recommendations the duration of treatment for different forms of IE and various bacteria is indicated, but patients are not alike. In our opinion determination of CRP is of value in the decision on the duration of IE treatment. When two normal CRP concentrations have been achieved, treatment was stopped. Only one of our 126 patients assessed had a relapse.

Treatment in this patient with late-onset PE due to *M. sedantarius* was discontinued after 92 days (6 years before an aortic conduit with an aortic valve was inserted), whilst CRP concentrations were still slightly elevated. Successful treatment of the relapse PE required 142 days.

Prevention of infective endocarditis

Antimicrobial prophylaxis

In spite of the lack of controlled studies and the lack of knowledge concerning its preventive efficacy, there is consensus that antimicrobial prophylaxis is indicated for patients with a valvular heart disease, small cardiac defects inducing jet streams or a prosthetic heart valve or conduits who undergo dental or medical procedures giving rise to bacteremia. However, about 50 percent of patients in whom IE develop, have normal or apparently normal hearts prior to illness [4] and less than 20 percent of the patients with viridans streptococcal endocarditis and only about 40 percent of the patients with enterococcal endocarditis had undergone procedures for which prophylaxis is recommended. In addition, approximately one quarter of the microorganisms causing IE are not susceptible to the antibiotics recommended for prophylaxis.

It has been calculated that less than 10 percent of cases with IE is prevented if there is a high compliance among patients and doctors for the recommended antimicrobial prophylaxis. Although prophylaxis will not influence the frequency of IE [4], morbidity linked to the occurrence of IE in particular patients will be less.

Former recommendations were rather complex. In addition parenteral administration of antibiotics encountered low compliance for the recommendations among patients as well as among doctors and dentists. Newer recommendations are simpler [34–36]. Oral high dose amoxycillin is given once or twice to cover the bacteremia induced by dental and upper respiratory tract procedures [34, 35]. Outside the hospital, patients at high risk because they have had a previous attack of IE, or because they have a cardiac prosthesis receive the same prophylaxis. In the USA this has been questioned. There the recommendations single out the particularly high risk patients for parental prophylaxis [36]. Compliance with the oral prophylaxis for IE seems to be rather high [34] providing the opportunity to lower the frequency of IE in known endocarditis prone patients.

Patients at risk undergoing surgery or instrumentation of the genitourinary tract or gastrointestinal tract should have appropriate prophylaxis, mostly amoxycillin in combination with gentamicin.

Cardiac surgery

Antimicrobial prophylaxis for open heart surgery is a well accepted practice despite the paucity of supportive data documenting its value. In 96 percent of operations for value repair or replacement and in 91 percent of coronary bypass operations antibiotic prophylaxis is given as reported recently in a study from the USA [37]. The length of the prophylaxis differs considerably among the different hospitals. In approximately 50 percent of the hospitals antibiotics are given for two days. A substantial number of patients receive prophylactic antibiotics for three to five days. Various antibiotics are used. In the USA most commonly first or second generation cephalosporins (80 percent of operations) are given just before and during surgery. Elsewhere flucloxacillin along or in combination with gentamicin is used [38]. Despite numerous trials comparing a variety of antimicrobial agents no clear conclusions can be drawn regarding the optimal choice.

Addendum

After this manuscript had been prepared an additional report has appeared about prevention of bacterial endocarditis. This report of Dajani et al. (JAMA 1990; 264: 2919–2922) is an update of the recommendations made in 1984 [36]. Standard prophylactic regimen for all dental, oral and upper respiratory tract procedures is amoxicillin (3 grams orally, 1 h before procedure; then 1.5 gram, 6 h initial dose). In addition, alternate prophylactic regimens are given for patients who are allergic to amoxicillin, for patients unable to take oral medications and patients considered high risk.

References

1. Kaye D. Definitions and demographic characteristics. In: Kay D, editor. Infective endocarditis. Baltimore: University Park Press, 1976:1–10.
2. Von Reyn CF, Levy BS, Arbeit RD, Friedland G, Crumpacker CS. Infective endocarditis: An analysis based on strict case definitions. Ann Intern Med 1981;94:505–18.
3. Kaye D. Changing pattern of infective endocarditis. Am J Medicine 1985;78 (Suppl 6B):157–62.
4. Bayliss R, Clarke C, Oakley C, Somerville W, Whitfield AGW. The teeth and infective endocarditis. Br Heart J 1983;50:506–12.
5. Scheld WM, Sande MA. Endocarditis and intravascular infections. In: Mandell GL, Douglas RG Jr, Bennett JE, editors. Principles and practice of infectious disease, 2nd ed., New York: John Wiley and Sons, 1985:504–30.
6. Rowley KM, Clubb KS, Smith GJW, Cabin HS. Right-sided infective endocarditis as a consequence of flow-directed pulmonary artery catheterization. A clinicopathological study of 55 autopsied patients. N Engl J Med 1984;311:1152–6.
7. Terpenning MS, Buggy BP, Kauffman CA. Hospital-acquired infective endocarditis. Arch Intern Med 1988;148:1601–3.
8. Terpenning MS, Buggy BP, Kauffman CA. Infective endocarditis; Clinical features in young and elderly patients. Am J Med 1987;83:626–34.
9. Pulliam L, Dall L, Inokuchi S, Wilson W, Hadley WK, Mills J. Effects of exopolysaccharide production by viridans streptococci on penicillin therapy of experimental endocarditis. J. Infect Dis 1985; 151:153–6.
10. Mayer KH, Schoenbaum SC. Evaluation and management of prosthetic valve endocarditis. Prog Cardiovasc Dis 1982;25:43–54.
11. Nihoyannopoulus P, Oakley CM, Exadactylos N, Ribeiro P, Westaby S, Foale RA. Duration of symptoms and the effects of a more aggressive surgical policy: Two factors affecting prognosis of infective endocarditis. Eur Heart J 1985;6:380–90.
12. Critten J, Waldvogel FA. Endocartides bactériennes: Aspects cliniques, bactériologiques et facteurs de prognostic. Schweiz Med Wochenschz 1977;107(Suppl 51):1–26.
13. Espersen F, Frimodt-Moller N. Staphylococcus aureus endocarditis. Arch Intern Med 1986;146:1118–21.
14. Daniel WG, Mügge A, Martin RP, et al. Improvement in the diagnosis of abscesses associated wih endocarditis by transesophageal echocardiography. N Eng J Med 1991;324:795–9.
15. Washington JA. The microbiological diagnosis of infective endocarditis. J Antimicrob Chemother 1987;20(Suppl A):29–36.
16. Werner AS, Cobbs CG, Kaye D, Hook EW. Studies on the bacteremia of bacterial endocarditis. J Am Med Assoc 1967;202:199–203.
17. Bayer AS. Staphylococcal bacteremia and endocarditis. State of the art. Arch Intern Med 1982;142:1169–77.
18. Bisno AL, Dismukes WE, Durack DT, et al. Antimicrobial treatment of infective endocarditis due to viridans streptococci, enterococci and staphylococci. J Am Med Assoc 1989;261:1471–7.
19. Report of a Working Party of the British Society for Antimicrobial Chemotherapy. Antibiotic treatment of streptococcal and staphylococcal endocarditis. Lancet 1985;2:815–7.
20. Drake TA, Sande MA. Antimicrobial treatment: Lessons from experimental models. In: Sande MA, Kaye D, Root RK, editors. Endocarditis. New York: Churchill Livingstone, 1984:77–100.
21. Scheld WM. Therapy of streptococcal endocarditis: Correlation of animal model and clinical studies. J Antimicrob Chemother 1987; 20(Suppl A): 271–85.
22. Wilson WR, Giuliani ER, Geraci JE. Treatment of penicillin-sensitive streptococcal infective endocarditis. Mayo Clin Proc 1982;57:45–50.
23. Meylan P, Francioli P, Glauser MP. Discrepancies between minimal bactericidal concentrations and actual killing of viridans group streptococci by cell-wall-active antibiotics. Antimicrob Agents Chemother 1986;29:418–22.

24. Wilson WR. Antimicrobial therapy of streptococcal endocarditis. J Antimicrob Chemother 1987;20(Suppl A):147–59.
25. Meeson J, McColm AA, Acred P, Greenwood D. Differential response to benzylpenicillin in vivo of tolerant and non-tolerant variants of Streptococcus sanguis II. J. Antimicrob Chemother 1990;25:103–9.
26. DiNubile M. Treatment of endocarditis caused by relatively resistant nonenterococcal streptococci. Is penicillin enough? Rev Infect Dis 1990;12:112–7.
27. Maki DG, Agger WA. Enteroccocal bacteremia, clinical features, the risk of endocarditis and management. Medicine 1988;67:248–69.
28. Eykin SJ. The treatment of staphylococcal endocarditis. J Antimicrob Chemother 1987;20 (Suppl A):161–7.
29. Cantoni L, Wenger A, Glauser MP, Bille J. Comparative efficacy of amoxycillin-clavulanate, cloxacillin and vancomycin against methicillin-sensitive and methicillin-resistant Staphylococcus aureus endocarditis in rats. J Infect Dis 1989;159:989–93.
30. Voorn GP, Thompson J, Goessens WHF, Schmal-Bauer W, Broeders PHM, Michel MF. Role of tolerance in cloxacillin treatment of experimental Staphylococcus aureus endocarditis. J Infect Dis 1991;163:640–3.
31. Eykyn SJ. The role of the laboratory in assisting treatment. A review of current UK practises. J Antimicrob Chemother 1987;20 (Suppl A):51–64.
32. Douglas A, Moore-Gillon J, Eykyn S. Fever during treatment of infective endocarditis. Lancet 1986;1:1341–3.
33. Kaye D. Prophylaxis for infective endocarditis: An update. Ann Intern Med 1986;104:419–23.
34. Shanson DC. Antibiotic prophylaxis of infective endocarditis in the United Kingdom and Europe. J Antimicrob Chemother 1987;20 (Suppl A):119–31.
35. Endocarditis Working Party of the British Society for Antimicrobial Chemotherapy. Antibiotic prophylaxis of infective endocarditis. Lancet 1990;1:88–9.
36. Shulman ST, Amren DP, Bisno AL, Dajani AS, Durack DT, Gerber M et al. Prevention of bacterial endocarditis: A statement for health professionals by the committee on rheumatic fever and infective endocarditis of the council on cardiovascular disease in the young. Circulation 1984;7:1123A–7A.
37. LoCicero J. Prophylactic antiobitic usage in cardio thoracic surgery. Chest 1990;98:719–23.
38. Editorial. Antibiotic cover for cardiac surgery. Lancet 1985;2:701–2.

13. Surgery for congenital heart disease in adults

A.J.J.C. BOGERS

Introduction

With increasing safety and effectiveness of cardiac surgery, an increasing number of adult patients with congenital heart disease becomes candidate for surgical correction [1, 2]. For some of these patients this is the first operation, because they have been asymptomatic or because the risk of surgery decreased below the gradually increasing risk of continued conservative treatment. For an increasingly important number of these patients this means a reoperation, the patient being a survivor of surgical therapy performed in infancy and childhood [1, 2].

In this last group of patients, residual (e.g. recoarctation of the aorta after coarctectomy [3, 4]), ongoing (e.g. right ventricular dysfunction after correction of tetralogy of Fallot [1, 2]), as well as newly developed problems (e.g. pulmonary valve regurgitation after transannular patching for tetralogy of Fallot [5]) may play a role in the indication for reoperation.

To demonstrate the diversity in diagnosis as well as surgical possibilities in the adult patients with congenital heart disease, recent experience is presented.

Materials and methods

All 82 patients of over 17 years of age, with congenital heart disease, registered to be operated in the Department of Thoracic Surgery of the Dijkzigt University Hospital from March 1988 to April 1991, are included in this report. Because 1 patient was operated twice, the study concerns 83 operations. The study includes 52 female and 30 male patients. Mean age was 38 years, range 18–75 years.

John Hess and George R. Sutherland (eds.), Congenital Heart Disease in Adolescents and Adults, 171–174.
© *1992 Kluwer Academic Publishers. Printed in the Netherlands.*

Results

The essential characteristics of the anatomic diagnosis of the 82 patients are recorded in Table 1.

Of the 83 operations 68 (82 percent) were primary operations and 15 (18 percent) were reoperations. Of the 68 primary operations, 64 were meant to be corrective and 4 were palliative (1 Fontanprocedure for tricuspid atresia, 1 Glennprocedure for tricuspid atresia, 1 debanding and Fontanprocedure for mitral atresia with ventriculoarterial discordance, 1 unifocalization procedure for pulmonary atresia with ventricular septal defect). The 15 reoperations were all after previous corrective surgery.

Table 1. Essentials of the anatomic diagnosis in adults operated for congenital heart disease in the Dijkzigt University Hospital from 3–88 to 4–91 (82 patients).

Sinus venosus defect	2
Secundum atrial septal defect	20
Atrial septal defect, valvular pulmonary stenosis	2
Morbus Ebstein	5
Tricuspid atresia	2
Mitral atresia, ventriculoarterial discordance	1
Partial atrioventricular septal defect	5
Complete atrioventricular septal defect	1
Ventricular septal defect	4
Ventricular septal defect, atrial septal defect	1
Double inlet left ventricle, subpulmonary stenosis	1
Tetralogy of Fallot	14
Subaortic stenosis	7
Subaortic stenosis, subpulmonary stenosis	1
Subpulmonary stenosis	2
Pulmonary atresia, ventricular septal defect	2
Valvular aortic stenosis, coarctation	1
Valvular pulmonary stenosis	1
Coronary arterial anomalies	4
Coarctation	6
Total	82

The 15 corrective reoperations were done in 14 patients. In 1 case, after previous closure of ventricular septal defect, a recurrent ventricular septal defect was directly closed. In 7 cases, after previous correction of tetralogy of Fallot, 8 reoperations were done. In 3 cases a recurrent ventricular septal defect was closed, in 2 with a prosthetic patch, in 1 by primary closure. In 1 case 2 recurrences of ventricular septal defect occurred and were closed in separate reoperations by prosthetic patch. In the 3 remaining cases, pulmonary regurgitation with right ventricular dysfunction was the most striking complication. In 1 case this was the only complication, which was treated by homograft pulmonary root replacement. In 1 case significant tricuspid regurgitation was present as well, the operation consisted of homograft pulmonary root replacement and tricuspid repair. In 1 case a recurrent ventricular septal defect was present as well, the operation consisted of homograft pulmonary root replacement and closure of the septal defect with a prosthetic patch. In 3 cases, after previous surgery for subaortic stenosis, recurrent subaortic stenosis was enucleated. In 3 cases, after previous surgery for coarctation, a recoarctation was treated by resection and end-to-end anastomosis in 2 of them and graft interposition in 1 case.

Hospital mortality concerned 3 patients (4 percent). A female patient of 22 years old, died 14 days after a primary and corrective operation for tetralogy of Fallot, due to multiple organ failure with sepsis and endocarditis, proven by autopsy. A female patient of 23 years old, died 2 days after corrective surgery for pulmonary atresia with ventricular septal defect, due to multiple organ failure with sepsis, proven by autopsy. A female patient of 34 years old, died 2 days after direct closure of a secundum atrial septal defect due to intractable ventricular arrhythmias.

Discussion

Recognition of the problem, organization of formal follow-up, centralization of the patients with informed cardiologists and surgeons, and knowledge including education, training and experience, are supposed to be vital in the solution of the problem of the adult patient with congenital heart disease [2]. Such prerequisites may be essential for an adequate appreciation of the wide variety in signs and symptoms caused by the adverse effects of the congenital heart defect on the myocardium and the cardiac function [6]. Consequently, cardiac surgery in these patients can be very complicated. This, as well as the importance of ongoing evaluation of longterm results of surgery for congenital heart disease, is well illustrated in the present series by the operations for subaortic stenosis and tetralogy of Fallot.

The 7 patients with subaortic stenosis include 3 patients being reoperated for recurrent subaortic stenosis. Until recently the mere finding of a discrete subaortic stenosis formed an indication for surgical therapy [7]. However, careful follow-up in our own series, revealed that both the natural history as well as the relapses in postsurgical history, are unpredictable in the seriousness and speed of progression of the subaortic stenosis [7]. This lead to a conservative change in indication for surgery for subaortic stenosis: in addition to the anatomic findings, progression to a significant gradient with signs of secondary left ventricular hypertrophy are now mandatory [7].

The 14 patients with 15 operations for tetralogy of Fallot are an example of the expanded surgical possibilities, due to the availability of homografts, for the reconstruction of the pulmonary outflow of the progressively overloaded right ventricle. In the 7 primary corrections the outflow tract was reconstructed by infundibulectomie in 2, by a transannular patch in 2 and with a homograft in 3. In the 3 reoperations in which pulmonary reconstruction was necessary, a homograft was used. It is noteworthy in this regard that arrhythmias can be the first or only symptom of the failing right ventricle and thus can form the indication for unloading the ventricle by implanting a functioning homograft between right ventricle and pulmonary artery.

In general, surgery for congenital cardiac defects, is a specialized field in which the surgeon requires experience in the repair of congenital defects allied to the skills of valve surgery, coronary grafting and reoperations [1]. In this regard, reentry to the heart needs careful assessment and planning, because adhesions are always present and contribute to the risk of bleeding. Moreover, patients can be at risk because of the presence of conduits or aneurysms or because of heart failure [8]. Depending on the indication for surgery, an alternative for resternotomy for cardiac reentry can be lateral thoracotomy [8]. Assessment of the route of reentry and specifically the retrosternal space, may include lateral X-rays, angiocardiograms, computerised tomography scanning and nuclear magnetic resonance [8]. Study of the reports of previous operations is essential [8]. Consequently the reentry should be performed by the responsible surgeon, who has to decide to what extent cardiopulmonary bypass should be standby or already in use (through femoral or iliac vessels) at reentry [8].

Consequently adult patients with congenital heart disease should be operated on in integrated surgical units where adult and congenital cardiac surgery are combined [1].

Taking this into account, primary surgery as well as reoperations in adults for congenital heart disease are highly feasable and can be performed with an acceptable risk.

References

1. Sutherland GR, Hess J, Roelandt J, Quaegebeur JM. The increasing problem of young adults with congenital heart disease. Eur Heart J 1990;11:4–6.
2. Somerville J. Grown-up survivors of congenital heart disease: Who knows? Who cares? Br J Hosp Med 1990;43:132–6.
3. Taylor JFN. Investigation before reoperations for congenital heart disease. In: Stark J, Pacifico AD, editors. Reoperations in cardiac surgery. London: Springer, 1989:3–16.
4. Kappetein AP. Surgical correction of coarctation of the aorta under the age of 3 years. Thesis, Leiden, 1991.
5. Pacifico AD. Reoperations after tetralogy of Fallot. In: Stark J, Pacifico AD, editors. Reoperations in cardiac surgery. London: Springer, 1989:171–83.
6. Bogers AJJC, van der Laarse A, Vliegen HW, et al. Assessment of hypertrophy in myocardial biopsies taken during correction of congenital heart disease. Thorac Cardiovasc Surg 1987;36:137–40.
7. de Vries A, Hess J, Witsenburg M, Frohn-Mulder IME, Bogers AJJC, Bos E. Management of fixed subaortic stenosis, a retrospective study in 57 patients. J Am Coll Cardiol 1992;19:1013–7.
8. Stark J. Approaches to the heart and great vessels at reoperation. In: Stark J, Pacifico AD, editors. Reoperations in cardiac surgery. London: Springer, 1989;43–53.

14. Cardiac transplantation for congenital heart disease in adolescents and adults

A.J.J.C. BOGERS & B. MOCHTAR

Introduction

Most patients with complex congenital heart malformations can be treated with some kind of palliative or (staged) corrective repair [3]. Only a small proportion of these patients do not reach definitive repair or the definitive repair has a very limited effect, because of inadequate chamber size, poor ventricular function, valvular dysfunction or high pulmonary vascular resistence [3]. Of this small proportion of patients in which further standard medical or surgical treatment is not possible, some patients can become candidate for cardiac transplantation.

In this setting, the treatment of the patients with otherwise incurable, end-stage congenital heart disease by cardiac transplantation, is being considered feasable in neonates and infants, and has become a rational therapy in adolescents and adults [4, 6, 8]. Already it is clear that, in the patient group that has received a heart transplant for congenital heart disease, accelerated graft atherosclerosis is also the limiting factor of long-term survival and a predominant cause of late death as well [4, 8, 10]. Accelerated graft sclerosis has been suggested to be more frequent in the pediatric age group than in the adult population [11]. The assumption that graft atherosclerosis is, at least in part, an immunological phenomenon, obviates the need for more adequate immunosuppressive treatment [2, 11].

Indications

For patients with congenital heart disease, the same criteria as for other heart disease are applied to become a possible candidate for cardiac transplantation [9]. The cardiac disease should be in an end-stage. The patient should be in functional class IV according to the New York Heart Association, despite

John Hess and George R. Sutherland (eds.), Congenital Heart Disease in Adolescents and Adults, 175–178.
© *1992 Kluwer Academic Publishers. Printed in the Netherlands.*

tailored medical therapy. There should be no other reasonable medical or surgical option available. The probability of survival should be less than 10 percent within 1 year without heart transplantation. Psychosocial stability and cooperation of the patient are as important as the medical conditon of the patient.

Limitations

Technically, cardiac transplantation is feasable even for the most complex lesions, except for those with an inadequate size of the pulmonary arteries [3]. In this regard techniques have been described for cardiac transplantation in situs abnormalities [11]. Anomalies of venous return and arterial outflow (i.e. ventriculoarterial discordancy) are also not necessarily a technical limit, provided that the recipient structures of concern are amply dissected and that ample length of donorstructures are procured [1, 3, 5, 11]. Baffle constructions for abnormalities of situs or venous return have been described [1, 11]. Previous palliative or reconstructive operations involving the pulmonary arterial system were reported not to be an obstacle for successful cardiac transplantation [1, 3, 5].

However, elevated pulmonary vascular resistence can be a contraindication to orthotopic cardiac transplantation, because this will lead to lethal failure of the right ventricle of the donor heart [3, 9, 11]. The physiologic upper limit of resistence within which orthotopic cardiac transplantation can successfully be done, has not exactly been determined. In adults a resistence of more than 6 units is accompanied with an increased risk of early mortality after transplantation, but in children successful transplantation has been reported with a pulmonary vascular resistence of up to 15 units [3]. Reversibility of the pulmonary vascular resistence of the recipient and the size of the donor heart should always be taken into account [3].

Considerations on hepatic function, renal function, systemic disease, malignancy, infection and trombo-embolic disease in the setting of cardiac transplantation, are the same for end-stage congenital heart disease as for other end-stage heart disease [3, 8, 11].

Inadequate psychosocial support that can complicate the intensive follow-up that is required for a patient after transplantation can be a contraindication to the procedure [3, 9, 11]. Although patients with congenital heart disease are experienced patients, prediction of behaviour after cardiac transplantation is difficult, especially in adolescents [3].

Shortage of appropriate donor hearts is a universal problem and affects patients with end-stage congenital heart disease as much as all other patients with end-stage cardiac disease.

Results

No series of cardiac transplantations exclusively for congenital heart disease have been reported, neither for neonates and infants, nor for adolescents and adults.

Nevertheless, heart transplantation in neonates and infants has been a rapidly growing area during the last years [7]. Consequently, congenital heart disease has surpassed cardiomyopathy as the primary indication for heart transplantation in the pediatric population since 1988 [7]. In our Rotterdam-Leiden-Nieuwegein series of 175 cardiac transplantations, only 2 adult patients were operated for end-stage congenital heart disease, see Table 1. Both patients are alive and well, 6 and 4 years after cardiac transplantation, respectively.

Table 1. Cardiac transplantation for congenital heart disease in the Rotterdam-Leiden-Nieuwegein series.

Anatomy	Age at operation	Follow-up
Patient 1: Dextrocardia Situs solitus Atrioventricular discordance Ventriculoarterial discordance	46 years	6 years
Patient 2: Situs inversus Atrioventricular discordance Ventriculoarterial discordance	33 years	4 years

Actuarial probability of survival for pediatric series, including transplantations for congenital as well as acquired cardiac disease, is reported to be 50–70 percent at 1 year and 40–65 percent at 2 years [6, 11].

Actuarial probability of survival in overall adult series is reported to be 82–89 percent at 1 year, 80–88 percent at 2 years and 78–88 percent at 3 years [9]. It seems reasonable to assume that results for cardiac transplantation in adolescents and adults for congenital heart disease, can be interposed between these results.

References

1. Allard M, Assaad A, Baily L., et al. Surgical techniques in pediatric heart transplantation. J Heart Lung Transplant 1991;10:808–27.
2. Balk AHMM, Simoons, ML, Jutte NHPM, et al. Sequential OKT3 and cyclosporine after heart transplantation: a randomized study with single and cyclic OKT3. Clin Transplant 1991;5:301–5.
3. Benson L, Freedom RM, Gersony W, Gundry R, Sauer U. Cardiac replacement in infants and children: Indications and limitations. J Heart Lung Transplant 1991;10:791–801.

4. Cooley DA Pediatric heart transplantation in historical perspective. J Heart Lung Transplant 1991;10:787–90.
5. Cooper MM, Fuzesi L, Addonizio LJ, Hsu DT, Smith CR, Rose EA. Pediatric heart transplantation after operations involving the pulmonary arteries. J Thorac Cardiovasc Surg 1991;102:386–95.
6. Hehrlein FW, Netz H, Moosdorf R, et al. Pediatric heart transplantation for congenital heart disease and cardiomyopathy. Ann Thorac Surg 1991;52:112–7.
7. Kriett JM, Kaye MP. The registry of the International Society of Heart and Lung Transplantation: Eighth official report – 1991. J Heart Lung Transplantation 1991;10:491–8.
8. Mill MR, Stinson EB. Heart and lung retransplantation. In: Stark J, Pacifico AD, editors. Reoperations in cardiac surgery. London: Springer, 1989:93–103.
9. Mochtar B. Medium term results in clinical orthotopic heart transplantation. Thesis, Rotterdam, 1991.
10. Pahl E, Fricker FJ, Armitage J, et al. Coronary arteriosclerosis in pediatric heart transplant survivors: Limitation of long-term survival. J Pediatr 1990;116:171–6.
11. Vouhé P. Transplantation of thoracic organs in children. In: Fallis JC, Miller RM, Lemoine G, editors. Pediatric thoracic surgery. New York: Elsevier, 1991:319–29.

15. Congenital heart disease in adolescents and adults: obstetric-gynaecologic counselling

FREDERIK K. LOTGERING

Introduction

Sex and childbearing are of great importance to young women and affect their life and happiness. To women with congenital heart disease the question 'conception or contraception?' may be even more vital, both from a somatic and psychologic point of view. The obstetric-gynecologic counsellor, in cooperation with the cardiologist, may help to reduce anxiety and assist the patient to reach a balanced decision. The variables pregnancy, disease, and treatment/medication affect each other as will be discussed below.

Pregnancy

Pregnancy is a process of adaptation which starts with conception, enables the development and growth of the conceptus within the mother, and ends with birth. Fertility nor the chance of spontaneous abortion are affected by maternal heart disease. However, the period of fetal growth and development requires marked maternal cardiovascular adaptations to meet the metabolic demands of the fetus and placenta. If these demands exceed the functional reserve of a pregnant cardiac patient, both the mother and the fetus are at risk. The circulatory changes during labor, delivery, and the postpartum period may impose an additional burden and further increase the risk of poor pregnancy outcome.

Fetoplacental metabolism accounts for an increase in overall metabolism of about 20 percent [1]. In response, uterine blood flow increases more than tenfold, to approximately 700 ml.min^{-1} near term [19, 20]. Probably mediated by this functional shunt and by placental hormones, maternal blood and plasma volumes increase during pregnancy by about 40 percent and 50 percent, respectively [7], and cardiac output increases by about 45 percent [2]. The

John Hess and George R. Sutherland (eds.), Congenital Heart Disease in Adolescents and Adults, 179–186.
© *1992 Kluwer Academic Publishers. Printed in the Netherlands.*

hemodynamic values as obtained in a recent study [2] of healthy women during the third trimester of pregnancy and twelve weeks postpartum are shown in Table 1. Cardiac output was found to be increased during pregnancy by 44 percent, from 4.3 to 6.2 l.min^{-1}, as a result of a 17 percent increase in heart rate, from 71 to 83 beats.min^{-1} and a 23 percent increase in stroke volume, from 61 to 75 ml. Systemic vascular resistance was calculated to be reduced by 21 percent, from 1530 to 1210 dyne.cm.sec^{-5}, and pulmonary vascular resistance by 34 percent, from 119 to 78 dyne.cm.sec^{-5}. Despite the increases in blood volume and venous return during pregnancy, no significant changes were observed in central venous pressure, pulmonary artery pressure, or pulmonary capillary wedge pressure. Mean arterial pressure, measured during the third trimester of pregnancy, in this study [2] was not different from the postpartum control value of 86 mmHg. Arterial pressure is approximately 15 percent lower during midgestation than it is near term whereas cardiac output increases early in gestation and remains at the same elevated level throughout pregnancy [20]. Consequently, systemic vascular resistance during midgestation must be approximately 15 percent lower than near term and 33 percent lower than in nonpregnant women, as has indeed recently been demonstrated (W. Visser and H.C.S. Wallenburg, personal communication).

Table 1. Normal hemodynamic changes during pregnancy.

	Near term pregnancy (36–38 weeks)	Postpartum control (12 weeks pp)	Pregnancy change (%)
Cardiac output (L. min^{-1})	6.2 ± 1.0	4.3 ± 0.9	44[a]
Heart rate (beats. min^{-1})	83 ± 10	71 ± 10	17[a]
Stroke volume (ml. beat^{-1})	75 ± ?	61 ± ?	23[a]
Central venous pressure (mmHg)	3.6 ± 2.5	3.7 ± 2.6	− 3
Mean arterial pressure (mmHg)	90 ± 6	86 ± 8	5
Pulmonary artery pressure (mmHg)	6.0 ± ?	6.4 ± ?	− 6
Systemic vascular resistance (dyne. cm. sec^{-5})	1210 ± 266	1530 ± 520	− 21[a]
Pulmonary vascular resistance (dyne. cm. sec^{-5})	78 ± 22	119 ± 47	− 34[a]
Pulmonary capillary wedge pressure (mmHg)	7.5 ± 1.8	6.3 ± 2.1	19[a]

Values are means ± SD; n = 10. Adapted from Clark et al. [2].
[a]p < 0.05.

In late pregnancy, cardiac output is markedly affected by body position. In the supine position cardiac output is on average about 15 percent lower than in the lateral position [18], but a much larger reduction develops in about 5 percent to 10 percent of pregnant women, as part of the supine hypotensive syndrome [4]. The reduction in cardiac output has been attributed to reduced venous return as a result of obstruction to flow in the inferior vena cava by the pregnant uterus [4]. The magnitude of the reduction in venous return and cardiac output is thought to depend on the level of obstruction [9], and the efficiency of venous collateral channels [4].

Physical activity increases cardiac output obviously also during pregnancy. In healthy individuals, maximal oxygen uptake is limited by muscle metabolism rather than by the circulatory system, and maximal heart rate and aerobic power, or physical fitness, are unaffected by pregnancy [10]. However, in pregnant cardiac patients exercise tolerance is likely to be reduced on a cardiovascular basis. In addition, the pregnancy-induced weight increases the burden of all weightbearing activities.

Rapid hemodynamic changes occur during delivery. When the uterine muscle contracts forcibly during labor contractions, uterine blood flow is reduced and cardiac output and arterial blood pressure are temporarily increased [18]. These changes are more pronounced in the supine than in the lateral position, with increases of 25 percent and 8 percent in blood pressure, respectively [18]. In addition, rapid changes in venous return during delivery can be caused by changes in venous return during delivery can be caused by changes in body position, the Valsalva maneuver during pushing, blood loss, and anesthesia. Therefore, cardiac patients require monitoring of both the mother and the fetus during this time and precautions should be taken to minimize volume changes [14]. These may include the careful administration of epidural anesthesia, assisted vaginal delivery, the use of oxytocin and, after delivery, of diuretics. The use of cesarean section should be limited to obstetric indications only [14].

If one compares the cardiovascular changes during pregnancy and delivery to the changes during exercise, pregnancy itself resembles exercise training in many respects [8], and delivery may be regarded as a superimposed exercise test. The postpartum period can then be regarded as a volume loading test. All are tolerated well by healthy pregnant women but women with congenital heart disease may not have enough functional reserve to adjust to these demands. Although one might postulate that exercise testing could provide valuable information about the functional reserve required for the adaptation to pregnancy and the stress of delivery, its predictive value with regard to pregnancy outcome has not been assessed.

Heart disease

Most women with congenital heart disease reach childbearing age either because they have an anomaly which is associated with long-term survival or because they have been successfully treated with cardiac surgery [12]. Because of this positive selection most pregnant patients will have enough functional reserve to tolerate pregnancy well.

Maternal mortality is significantly increased and pregnancy is contraindicated, however, in cases associated with severe pulmonary hypertension and/or right-to-left shunt, including Eisenmenger syndrome and Tetralogy of Fallot, and in cases with an increased risk of aortic rupture, like complicated Marfan syndrome and aortic coarctation [12, 14, 15]. The pregnancy-induced increase in cardiac output and the reduction in systemic vascular resistance will enhance shunting and cyanosis in the first group. Eisenmenger syndrome is associated with approximately 50 percent maternal mortality [15] and is therefore considered one of the few valid indications for therapeutic abortion. In untreated cases of Tetralogy of Fallot mortality may be as high as 7 percent, whereas outcome in surgically corrected cases is generally good. In Marfan's syndrome the hyperdynamic circulation in pregnancy is held responsible for the maternal mortality which may be as high as 50 percent if significant annuloaortic ectasia is present [12, 15], but is uneventful in most other cases. The present functional cardiac status is of greater importance than the original lesion, as maternal mortality varies directly with NYHA functional class [12], and prognosis is poor in cyanotic disease [15].

Fetal outcome is also affected by maternal functional class as fetal mortality varies from nil in class I to 30 percent in class IV patients [12]. This has been attributed to the fact that prematurity and dysmaturity are common in women with cyanotic heart disease, probably as a result of fetal hypoxia [12]. In addition, congenital heart disease of the mother increases considerably the risk of heart disease in the fetus. Empiric risk figures vary from 3 percent for Tetralogy of Fallot to 18 percent for aortic stenosis [5, 14, 17]. The value of genetic counselling of patients with congenital heart defects has been considered elsewhere in this book. The most important practical consequence of the high risk figures is the need for fetal echocardiography during pregnancy. In experienced hands, the presence or absence of a congenital heart defect in the fetus can be accurately detected with the use of echocardiography from a gestational age of about 18 weeks [17]. In the few cases in which the congenital heart defect is likely to be incompatible with postnatal survival, the parents may wish to consider abortion or to abstain from obstetric intervention in case of fetal distress during labor. In less severe cases, parents and physicians may anticipate neonatal evaluation and treatment. Most importantly, fetal echocardiography may help to reduce anxiety in the majority of patients, by the reassuring finding that their unborn child does not have a detectable heart defect [17].

Treatment

Maternal interests must always prevail over fetal concerns. Therefore, if maternal heart disease requires treatment during pregnancy fetal side effects are of secondary importance. Nonetheless, it is good to realize that maternal treament may markedly affect fetal well-being. Cardiac surgery during pregnancy, for example, is associated with a fetal mortality of 30 percent [12], and most drugs readily cross the placenta. Therefore, if functional reserve can be improved by surgery it should preferably be performed prior to conception rather than during pregnancy. Of the commonly used drugs, coumarins have been demonstrated to cause fetal anomalies, especially when they were administered during the first trimester of pregnancy. Therefore, they should be replaced by heparin before or soon after conception [6]. Coumarins should also be replaced by heparin near term, or when delivery is imminent, in order to avoid maternal and fetal hemorrhage. Other cardiovascular drugs do not have equally evident fetal side effects. However, most drugs have not been studied well enough to exclude the possibility of adverse effects on the fetus or neonate. Among the drugs that are likely to have an undesired pharmacologic effect on the fetus are the adrenergic agent propanolol and the anticholinergic agents atropin and scopalamin [13]. Among the relatively safe drugs are the antiarrythmic lidocaine and the diuretic thiazides [6]. Among the antihypertensive drugs, alpha-methyldopa has been most widely used during pregnancy to treat preexisting hypertension, and hydralazine to treat acute increases in blood pressure associated with preeclampsia. Both are considered to be fairly safe [6]. In contrast, the antihypertensive drug labetalol has recently been scutinized for its use in severe preeclampsia, because its combined alpha-beta-blocking effect may persist in the neonate and be life threatening (W. Visser and H.C.S. Wallenburg, personal communication). One should realize that all antihypertensive drugs tend to reduce uterine perfusion pressure and, because the uterine vascular bed lacks autoregulation [19], also uterine blood flow. Therefore, antihypertensive drugs may jeopardize fetal oxygenation and well-being.

Antibiotics are widely used in the prophylactic treatment of women with congenital heart disease in labor. One should realize, however, that the risk of bacterial endocarditis is low with vaginal delivery, that the liberal use of antibiotics is not without risk, and that the efficacy of prophylactic antibiotic treatment in parturient women has not been demonstrated.

Contraception

Sexual activity itself carries definable risks and only abstinence imparts zero risk. This fact is often overlooked [3]. The main risks are sexually transmitted diseases and unwanted pregnancy. The prevention of sexually transmitted disease is beyond the scope of this review. Unwanted pregnancy can be prevented by contraceptive methods or treated by abortion. One should realize that prevention is better than to cure, and that abortion is not a contraceptive method.

All contraceptive methods have their own inherent risks. Yet, most women with congenital heart disease do require some kind of contraception during most of their reproductive life. In each individual case the decision either to use, or not to use, contraception should be based on a calculation of risks and benefits. Because sexual behaviour is stronger than tabu, consultation should start at an early age, preferably at the onset of puberty.

Of the available methods, low dose oral contraceptives must be considered first choise in most cases. Oral contraceptives have been studied most extensively, are effective, and have few side effects. They are presently used by approximately 6.10^7 women worldwide [3]. The fact that oral contraceptive use imparts less overall risk to life than not using any form of contraception in women under 30 years of age and in nonsmokers through age 40, has led to nonprescription availability in many countries [3].

The most important health concern associated with the use of oral contraceptives is the consistently higher incidence of thromboembolism observed in case control and cohort studies, with relative risk figures varying between 3 and 12, but mortality statistics offer little support for a relationship between oral contraceptive use and cardiovascular events [16]. The risk of thromboembolic episodes increases with the estrogen dosage [11] and is approximately 4 per 1000 women years for those contraceptives containing 50 μg ethinylestradiol [11]. This has led to the development of lower dose estrogen contraceptives in recent years. Oral contraceptives have also been associated with hypertension and myocardial infarction, but the association is not very consistent [16]. These risks have been attributed to the progestogenic component [3] and this has led to recent modifications also in this component. Although the relative risk associated with the new low-dose oral contraceptives has yet to be established, it seems likely that the new generation of oral contraceptives does not predispose to thromboembolism or hypertension to the same extent as the older higher-dose preparations.

Most women with congenital heart disease are not at a markedly increased risk for thromboembolism and can safely use oral contraceptives. Oral contraceptives can also be prescribed without hesitation to those women who were at increased risk for thromboembolism but are on permanent anticoagulant therapy. Indeed, the use of oral contraceptives in these women has the advantage that it reduces the risks of excessive menstrual blood loss and ovulation bleeding. Women who do have an increased risk for thromboembolism should consider other contraceptive methods.

The intrauterine contraceptive device is generally considered the second best nonpermanent contraceptive method. It has a slightly higher pregnancy rate than the oral contraceptives and may increase the risk of pelvic infectious disease, notably in those women with more than one sexual partner. It is therefore relatively contraindicated in women at risk for bacterial endocarditis. Because menstrual blood loss is generally more pronounced, the intrauterine contraceptive device is also less suitable for women on anticoagulant therapy.

The barrier methods of contraception, condom and pessary, are cumbersome and less effective than the previous two methods and, therefore, less well accepted. However, they offer protection against sexually trasmitted disease and may be safe if used in combination with a sperm killing drug.

A woman may wish permanent contraception. Sterilization of the female is performed by occlusion of the Fallopian tube. It is an effective and relatively simple surgical procedure that is most commonly performed through the laparoscope under general anesthesia. In a monogamous relation vasectomy of the partner is equally effective and has the advantage of even simpler technique and local anesthesia. When both partners consider the family complete sterilization can be a satisfactory solution. However, if a woman demands sterilization for other reasons, such as fear, doctor's advice, or social circumstances, she may well regret the decision at a later point in time, especially if the procedure is performed at an early age or in association with an abortion. Therefore, sterilization should not be advised or performed easily, even in those women with severe congenital heart disease in which pregnancy is considered to be contraindicated.

Summary

To summarize, early ob/gyn counselling may help to reduce anxiety and uncertainty in those women with congenital heart disease who desire to become pregnant at some time in their life. In addition, it may help to prevent unwanted pregnancy and the need for elective abortion. Although pregnancy will require extra precautions, especially in the peripartum period, maternal and fetal outcome is generally good in women with congenital heart disease. Almost never will maternal health concerns justify the termination of pregnancy.

References

1. Clapp JF. Cardiac output and uterine blood flow in the pregnant ewe. Am J Obstet Gynecol 1978;130:419–23.
2. Clark SL, Cotton DB, Lee W, et al. Central hemodynamic assessment of normal human pregnancy. Am J Obstet Gynecol 1989;161:1439–42.
3. Derman R. Oral contraceptives: A reassessment. Obstet Gynecol Survey 1989;44:662–8.
4. Kerr MG. The mechanical effects of the gravid uterus in late pregnancy. J Obstet Gynecol Br Commonw 1965;72:513–29.
5. Lin AE, Garver KL. Genetic counselling for congenital heart defects. J Pediatr 1988;113:1105–9.
6. Little BB, Gilstrap LC. Cardiovascular drugs during pregnancy. Clin Obstet Gynecol 1989;32:13–20.
7. Longo LD. Maternal blood volume and cardiac output during pregnancy: A hypothesis of endocrinologic control. Am J Physiol 1983;245:R720–9.
8. Lotgering FK, Longo LD, Gilbert, RD. Maternal and fetal effects of exercise. Physiol Rev 1985;65:1–36.
9. Lotgering FK, Wallenburg HCS. Hemodynamic effects of caval and uterine venous occlusion in pregnant sheep. Am J Obstet Gynecol 1986;155:1164–70.
10. Lotgering FK, van Doorn MB, Struijk PC, Pool J, Wallenburg HCS. Maximal aerobic exercise in pregnant women: Heart rate, O_2 consumption, CO_2 production, and ventilation. J Appl Physiol 1991;70:1016–23.
11. Meade TW. Risks and mechanisms of cardiovascular events in users of oral contraceptives. Am J Obstet Gynecol 1988;158:1646–52.

12. Perloff JK. Congenital heart diseases and pregnancy. In: Gleicher N, editor. Principles of medical therapy in pregnancy. New York: Plenum, 1985:665–71.

13. Piper JM, Baum C, Kennedy DL, Price P. Maternal use of prescribed drugs associated with recognized fetal adverse drug reactions. Am J Obstet Gynecol 1988;159:1173–7.

14. Pitkin RM, Perloff JK, Koos BJ, Beall MH. Pregnancy and congenital heart disease. Ann Int Med 1990;112:445–54.

15. Ramin S, Maberry MC, Gilstrap LC. Congenital heart disease. Clin Obstet Gynecol 1989;32:41–7.

16. Realini JP, Goldzieher JW. Oral contraceptives and cardiovascular disease: A critique of the epidemiologic studies. Am J Obstet Gynecol 1985;152:729–98.

17. Stewart PA. Echocardiography in the human fetus. Doctoral thesis, Erasmus University Rotterdam, 1989.

18. Ueland K, Hausen JM. Maternal cardiovascular dynamics. II. Posture and uterine contractions. Am J Obstet Gynecol 1969;103:1–7.

19. Wallenburg HCS. Modulation and regulation of utero-placental blood flow. Placenta 1981;(suppl 1): 45–64.

20. Wallenburg HCS. Maternal haemodynamics in pregnancy. Fetal Med Rev 1990;2:45–66.

21. Whittemore R. Genetic counseling for young adults who have a congenital heart defect. Pediatr 1986;13:220–7.

16. Psychosocial aspects of congenital heart disease in adolescents and adults

ELISABETH M.W.J. UTENS & RUDOLPH A.M. ERDMAN

From the early days of pediatric cardiac surgery several scientific publications have appeared concerning psychosocial aspects of congenital heart disease, further called CHD. In the Sixties and Seventies most of the studies attempted to describe the impact of CHD on family life [1–3]. Over the last 25 years advances in cardiovascular surgical techniques have reduced mortality and (pediatric) cardiologists are now faced with a growing population of adolescents and adults with corrected or modified congenital heart defects whose medical and personal needs are relatively unfamiliar, complex and challenging [4, 5].

This chapter is divided into three parts. In the first part attention will be paid to the influence of CHD on physical, emotional, cognitive and social functioning in children, adolescents and young adults as described in the literature. In this part results from early empirical studies as well as psychosocial findings derived from clinical practice will be described. The empirical studies, executed in the sixties and seventies, usually contained methodological flaws such as use of non-standardized interviews and observations of parents of sick infants and young children. The psychosocial findings, derived from clinical-therapeutic publications, need to be validated by empirical research. In short, the psychosocial aspects mentioned in the first part of this chapter need to be further investigated by means of standardized and reliable research. In the second part the results of two recently performed empirical follow-up studies will be reviewed in which social aspects and intellectual functioning of adolescents and adults have been studied. Finally, in the last part, the methodological design of the Rotterdam Follow-up Study on Quality of Life in CHD patients will be outlined. This follow-up study which was started in 1989 is financially supported by the Dutch Heart Foundation.

John Hess and George R. Sutherland (eds.), Congenital Heart Disease in Adolescents and Adults, 187–197.
© 1992 *Kluwer Academic Publishers. Printed in the Netherlands.*

Physical, emotional, cognitive and social aspects of CHD

In view of the diagnostic differences between congenital heart defects and between operated versus non-operated patients it is not possible to describe THE patient with CHD. Therefore, in this chapter a short review will be given of psychosocial aspects mentioned in the literature concerning adolescent and adult patients with CHD in general. Although many adolescents and young adults with CHD appear to be functioning well [6], the focus of this chapter will be on the potential psychosocial difficulties of CHD, since it is important that these are known to (pediatric) cadiologists.

Physical aspects

CHD can cause retardation in physical development. Linde et al. and Linde notice that in children with CHD growth retardation may be present, which is more marked for weight than for height and which is more prominent in those with cyanosis [7, 8]. Children with cyanotic CHD may show delayed pubescence. Varnauskas et al. [9] report that boys are more affected in growth than girls, especially in their second decade. However, most children with mild cardiac defects will grow normally. Physical retardation can result in the inability to participate in athletics or sports. According to Varnauskas et al. [9] children with growth retardation tend to be treated as younger than their chronologic age and they are frequently teased by their peer group. These aspects may lead to a diminished self-esteem and/or social isolation.

Correction of the cardiovascular abnormality usually results in an increase of the growth rate to normal dimensions. Although cardiac surgery has become increasingly safe and effective many adolescents and young adults have significant residual abnormalities, which may present major physical and/or psychological problems for the patient's future life [5]. As for working capacity Varnauskas et al. [9] describe that, despite favourable improvements after surgery, many postoperative patients have a functional capacity of 30–40 percent below the established normal values. To what extent this reduction in working capacity after successful surgery may be related to inadequate development and training of the cardiovascular system or to psychological factors (such as persistent parental overprotection) is an open question.

Emotional aspects

From the moment the physician's diagnosis of CHD is known, it does not only influence the afflicted child but also the family interrelations. The emotional development of the child with CHD may be hampered by parental attitudes, such as pampering and overprotection, and by maternal anxiety [4, 7, 10, 11]. Poor emotional adjustment of the afflicted child relates more to maternal anxiety and pampering than to the degree of incapacity or severity of disease

[8]. Maternal anxiety appears to be primarily a function of the presence of CHD itself rather than its severity [12]. With adequate parents however, most children with CHD find themselves well integrated in the family [4]. At schoolage, issues such as school activities, friendship and social activities can give rise to experiences of failure and ostracism. With growth to adolescence, these negative experiences are often confirmed and adolescents with ongoing CHD may cope poorly when confronted with problems and exhibit self-destructive tendencies, sadness, depression and loneliness. While parents may feel increasingly ambivalent, adolescents may experience confusion, guilt and rage [4]. They are often angry and confused about why they had to be born with CHD [4, 10]. Both patients and their families may experience a constant fear of sudden death and many adolescents fear they will not live past the age of 35 years [4].

The major developmental tasks of adolescence include adjusting to bodily changes, separation from parents and developing (sexual) identity. Because adolescents with CHD are capable of seeing the long-term consequences of illness, they are often preoccupied with their illness. Concerns often center on restrictions of CHD on social life, peer acceptance, identity issues and fears about the future [10]. Adolescents and young adults with CHD may experience greater uncertainty, vulnerability or feelings of inferiority than their healthy agemates, due to a number of factors, such as: their body concept; the scar; job hunting; courtship/marriage; intercourse; (anti-) conception.

According to Donovan and Garson and Baer [4, 6], adolescents and adults with CHD are at risk for developing a poor body concept and a preoccupation with and over-interpretation of body sensations. Many of these adolescents are particularly sensitive to being small or skinny and the over-interpretation of body sensations occasionally leads to hypochondria. Feelings of shame about the scar may arise when sexual advances are within reach. Conflicts may arise for adolescents and young adults when potential employers ask for a health history or require a medical examination and when they feel restricted because of physical limits. Rejection for the Army – for boys – may arouse feelings of worthlessness. Anxiety tends to be greater and conflicts sharper when courtship, intercourse and sexual arousal for boys and (anti)conception for girls come within reach. Young males with CHD may ask themselves whether strong sexual excitement can result in a myocardial infarction. Young females with CHD are sometimes concerned about whether oral anticonception can result in hypertension and harm the cardiovascular functioning. Young adults with CHD are very often afraid that they will pass their congenital defect to their offspring and young women are concerned about whether their heart is strong enough to sustain the labour in giving birth to a baby.

Adolescents and young adults with CHD may use a number of behavioural and cognitive strategies to cope with their stress, such as withdrawal from contacts, childish behaviour, denial, intellectualization and overcompensation [4, 6, 10]. Acting-out behaviour, such as refusal to cooperate with medical procedures or manipulation, are common reactions. Hospitalizations elicit regressive behaviour and in such circumstances adolescents need the presence and love of their parents. It is important to realize that the adolescent lives in a world full of conflicts: he is striving for a sense of independence while at the same time he needs his parents intensively [10].

Cognitive and intellectual aspects

In the pre-school period cognitive skills such as intelligence, long and short-term memory, the ability to concentrate and the integrative functions are still immature. Consequently for the young child it is absolutely impossible to understand why medical treatment and hospital admissions are necessary. Magic associative thinking combined with an egocentric and restricted comprehension of the world support the idea that medical treatment and hospitalization are to be considered a punishment for forbidden phantasies and misbehaviour. During the elementary school phase experienced pain is often considered a punishment and the child may have worrying thoughts about an early death [10]. Such kinds of thoughts are reinforced by a lack of or insufficient education. According to Brodie [13] chronically ill and frequently hospitalized children suffer from anxiety about their illness, have more knowledge about their illness and tend to view it more as punishment than healthy children do. Adolescents with CHD are often preoccupied with physical and technical information supply about their illness, which they may consider a punishment for forbidden phantasies or sexual activities [4, 10]. Because their perception of illness can be distorted, they may react more significantly to visible symptoms than to a life-threatening condition [10].

Parents of children with CHD are often concerned and anxious about possible deleterious effects of implied suboptimal cerebral oxygen supply on intellectual functioning. Research findings dated from the end of the Sixties showed that children with CHD scored lower on intelligence tests than normal children. The lower scores were particularly evident in the first three years of life and were more marked in cyanotic children [7, 8]. However, as Linde points out, the methods used to measure the intelligence levels in young children were inadequate since they relied heavily on gross motor functioning [8]. Because children with CHD may have impaired physical capacity that limits their ability to perform well on such tests, Linde [8] suggests that in these children a better estimate of intellectual capacity may be obtained from adaptive and social behaviour. For older children with CHD – for cyanotic as well as for acyanotic children – IQ scores within the normal range were found although their mean scores tended to fall in the lower end of the range of normal intelligence [7, 8].

After having reviewed the literature, Kitchen [12] reports that investigations into the possible relationship between intellectual functioning and CHD have yielded conflicting results. She reaches the tentative conclusion that – although low scores have been recorded in some afflicted children (both pre and postoperatively):

1. there does not exist a consistent relation between CHD (regardless of hemodynamic severity) and cognitive functioning; and that
2. hypothermic open heart surgery does not necessarily have long-term effects on intelligence levels.

Besides, she underlines that in future studies more explicit attention must be paid to other organic factors that might influence the intellectual functioning of CHD-children, such as coexisting developmental abnormalities of the brain. Further, intellectual functioning may be harmed by altered or limited environmental experiences such as school absence because of (cardiac) illness, parental patterns of absenting their child from school for minor illnesses, repeated hospital admissions and consequently decreased social contacts [8, 14]. During the last decade some follow-up studies into intellectual functioning have been executed, the samples of which mostly consisted of children younger than 10 years of age [15–18]. Later in this chapter, attention will be paid to a recent follow-up study on this subject, in which young adults with CHD participated.

Social aspects

In the preceding paragraphs some social aspects related to CHD have already been mentioned. Now further attention will be paid to the possible influence of CHD on situations at home, at school, at the labour sphere of action, at leisure-time activities and making and sustaining social contacts. Maxwell and Gane [1] investigated the impact of CHD upon family life with the help of a skilled social worker, who administered a questionnaire to 150 families with one thing in common: a child with inborn heart disease. Fifty-nine percent of the parents experienced some problems in rearing the affected child; mostly (in 50 percent of them) these were difficulties in disciplining the child and feeding difficulties were reported in 20 percent of them. Forty-three percent of the parents answered that 'spoiling' of the afflicted child occurred and 14 percent of these children appeared to share the parental bed, even though adequate accommodation was available. This last result may reflect continuing anxiety within the family. 'Checking at night' occurred in 64 percent of the families and in 10 percent this occurred over several years. Thirty-two percent of the families believed that the child might suddenly die. In 38 percent of the families the siblings had been affected in some way by the cardiac disease; in 18 percent of these families 'worry' in the siblings occurred, in 10 percent 'hostility' to and 'jealousy' of the afflicted child and in 3.2 percent 'deprivation feelings' in the siblings were reported. In 18 percent of the families the mutual relationship between the parents appeared to have deteriorated because of the cardiac disease. A total inability to adjust or accept at any level was found in 14 percent of these families. So far the results from this early study.

In 1983 Silverman [19] underlined that families of a child with CHD typically responded initially with shock and guilt, manifested by a stated inability to comprehend even the most simple explanations or to cope with child care at home. Further he made clear that variety in the adaptation process is rarely a function of educational level or social class. The crucial factor in the adaptation process appeared to be the state of the child's medical situation. According to Silverman [19] parents are often placed in the conflicting situation of offering all possible attention to their child after surgery and his return home versus the perceived need to avoid 'spoiling' the child and they are concerned about the possible detrimental effects of 'over-attention' of the afflicted child on other siblings and upon their marital relationship.

As for school functioning, irregular school attendance may turn the child or adolescent with CHD into an 'exceptional case' in the eyes of classmates, which may harm social contacts in class. This problem also arises when the child or adolescent cannot fully participate in gymnastics or is treated in a more careful way by teachers than classmates. Children and adolescents with cyanotic heart disease may become socially isolated because of their growth retardation, blueness or clubbed fingers. Restricted leisure-time activities, due to physical incapacity and/or parental overprotection, strengthen their social isolation. For some children with CHD, special and more individually oriented education may be required because of learning- or concentration difficulties. In schools for special education contacts with classmates may be facilitated. However, when such a school is not situated in the direct neighbourhood of the child's home, this may lead to practical difficulties as for sharing leisure time with friends from school. Further, the child with CHD may alienate from peers in the neighbourhood because of attending this special school. And as Bowen [10] reported 'rejection by a peer can be devastating'.

Problems concerning job hunting, courtship and marriage have been mentioned before. In 1983 Ghisla et al [20] reported that adolescents and adults with CHD were strongly limited in choosing the profession they wanted. However, the majority appeared to be satisfied with their profession of 'second-choice' and perceived their chances to make career at work as normal. As for courtship and marriage Donovan [4] stated that adolescents and adults are often confronted with in-law rejection. Further, they frequently have to face difficulties with pensions, health and life insurances, such as ineligibility or financial rates which are higher than for their normally healthy peers [4, 20]. In 1983 Silverman underlined that reliable data concerning the long-term social impact of (treatment of) CHD on teenagers and young adults is lacking [19].

Recent follow-up studies into psychosocial aspects of adolescents and adults with CHD

In the last decade some follow-up studies into psychosocial functioning of adolescents and adults with CHD have been executed, which cover a wide range of variables measured, such as: educational- and intellectual level, school absence, gymnastics and sports, military service, choice of profession and work experiences, medical examinations, insurances, leisure-time activities, marital status, pregnancies and number of offspring, psychological wellbeing, self-esteem and subjective evaluation of physical health. Most of the follow-up studies contained methodological weaknesses, such as use of small and hetero-geneous samples (e.g. patients with different diagnoses, combinations of ope-rated and non-operated, cyanotic and acyanotic patients) [14, 20–22]. Further, inadequate and weakly standardized test instruments were mostly used. Since it would go too far to review all studies, the follow-up studies done by Otterstad et al. [23] and by Jedlicka-Köhler and Wimmer [24] are selected to be described here for the following reasons. The study of Otterstad et al. [23] was chosen because in this study a differentiation was made between diagnostic groups. Besides, the mean age of the total sample was about 42 years whereas in other psychosocial follow-up studies (much) younger study populations were used. The study of Jedlicka-Köhler and Wimmer [24] was selected because it was the only follow-up study known to the authors, in which a group of young adults with CHD underwent standardized intelligence tests. Further, a clear differentiation was made between two groups of 'late' and 'early' operated patients.

The first is a study conducted in 1986 in Norway by Otterstad et al. [23], who investigated possible long-term deterioration of social functioning in adults over 30 years of age with congenital, isolated ventricular septum defects (VSD). The investigators assumed that deterioration might possibly have been caused by brain damage connected with open heart surgery performed after the age of 10. Thirty-five patients, who had undergone surgical repair of VSD at a mean age of 23 years (range: 10–51 years), were followed up for an average of 15 years (range: 3–21 years). Their mean age at time of restudy was 39 years (range: 31–61 years). These operated patients were called group I. Their social functioning was compared with 61 non-operated VSD patients with basically smaller defects, mean age 43 years (range: 31–73 years), who were followed up for an average of 14 years (range: 3–21 years). Data was gathered by means of a social medical questionnaire, the validity and reliability of which was not indicated. The non-operated patients were called group II. The results showed a statistically significant, subjective improvement in physical capacity at restudy among operated patients versus non-operated patients (p < 0.01). Moderate, unspecific symp-toms such as anxiety, atypical chest pain and dyspnoea, not related to physical exercise, were reported frequently in both groups (46 percent and 44 percent in groups I and II, respectively) and about 60 percent in both groups related them to the presence of the heart defect. In both groups normal social activities were reported by 90 percent. Both groups had a higher educational level than normal 40-year old Norwegians, insignificantly favouring group I. Similar proportions among both groups had physically heavy versus light work and similar proportions had obtained a disability pension. Regular medical check-ups were attended by 45 percent and 60 percent in group I and II, respectively. In group I slightly less mental stress at work and a moderately higher gross income were reported, although the differences were not statistically significant. Approximately 25 percent in both groups reported their heart defect as having had a negative influence on their freedom of choice of education and profession. The authors concluded that the operated patients had suffered no detrimental effects on their social function compared with the non-operated group. Therefore they advocated a liberal policy for surgical repair of VSD after the age of 10 years.

In 1987 Jedlicka-Köhler and Wimmer [24] published the results of a study regarding the influence of the time of operation on the intellectual and psychosocial development in children with Tetralogy of Fallot. The intention was to investigate to what extent the duration of chronic hypoxemia might influence intellectual and social development. Twenty four children underwent standardized intelligence tests and psychological questionnaires. Thirteen of them had had surgery in early infancy at a mean age of one year and seven months and at follow-up their mean age was 6 years and 5 months. The late operation group consisted of 11 children, who had a mean age of 8 years and 1 month at the time of surgery and of 18 years and 11 months at follow-up. No differences on intellectual level were found between both study groups. All 24 patients scored within the normal range of intellectual functioning. However, Jedlicka-Köhler and Wimmer concluded from their study that early surgery does appear to improve the social situation because children operated earlier participated in kindergarten and started elementary school in time more frequently and also passed through school without delay more often than children operated later. These results suggest a possible beneficial relief of the stressed situation for the whole family [24].

In general it can be concluded that follow-up studies on psychosocial functioning of adolescents and adults with CHD have yielded interesting but also confusing results up till now. In view of these puzzling results and of the methodological weaknesses mentioned above, one can only conclude that more and above all more systematized and multidisciplinary research still needs to be done. Sutherland et al. [5] underline that close follow-up of this new and expanding patient population is essential, as they are the first generation of survivors of surgical repair of CHD and many questions on their long-term future have yet to be answered. Baer et al. [25] point out that still relatively little is known about long-term psychological sequelae of childhood illnesses. A crucial and unsolved issue is whether surgical repair of CHD during childhood results in identifiable and predictable psychological consequences in adulthood and whether the nature of these psychological consequences is influenced by the age of the child at the time of surgical repair. To investigate this question among others, the following study was started in Rotterdam, the Netherlands.

Rotterdam Follow-Up Study on Quality of Life in children, adolescents and adults with surgical repair of CHD

In 1989 a follow-up study was started in the University Hospital Rotterdam to assess the quality of life (in a medical as well as in a psychological sense) at least nine years or longer after surgical correction for CHD in childhood. The main questions of this multidisciplinary study, carried out by a pediatric cardiologist and a clinical psychologist, are as follows:

1. Are adolescents and adults with operated CHD able to have a normal and satisfactory life with regard to physical exertion, stamina and muscular strength?
2. To what extent do they suffer residual cardiac symptoms?
3. Are there problems concerning intellectual, social and/or emotional development?
4. Is there any relationship between the original cardiologic anomaly and the current somatic condition and psychosocial functioning?

This study involves all patients who underwent (their first) cardiac surgery for CHD between 1968 and 1980 in the University Hospital Rotterdam and were younger than 15 years of age at the time of operation, a total of 712 patients. The ages range from 9 to 35 years. Within the study population a differentiation is made between 5 diagnostic groups: atriumseptum defect, ventricular septum defect, tetralogy of Fallot, transposition of the great arteries and a miscellaneous group. At follow-up 102 patients had died and 41 were lost to follow-up because they had moved abroad or because they were untraceable. Of the remaining 569 patients, 70 did not participate for various reasons. The final study population consists of 499 participants. The response rate, corrected for deceased patients and persons lost to follow-up, is 87.7%. The age distribution of the study population is shown in Table 1.

Table 1. Age distribution of the study population of the Rotterdam Follow-Up Study on Quality of Life in CHD patients.

9–10 years: N = 24	N = 149	
11–15 years: N = 125		N = 499
16–17 years: N = 61	N = 350	
18–35 years: N = 289		

In Table 2 a summary is given of the psychosocial variables, which are measured in the study population by means of psychological questionnaires – tests and semi-structured interviews. Most of the psychosocial parameters have been standardized at a national or international level. The parents of children younger than 16 years of age, are also interviewed and are requested to fill out several psychological questionnaires with respect to the behaviour of the child.

Table 2. Psychosocial variables measured in the Rotterdam Follow-up Study on Quality of Life in CHD patients.

Biographical variables:	Family constellation, socio-economical status and religion of parents.
Intermediating variables:	Life events.
Emotional variables:	Emotional- and behavioural problems, psychological wellbeing, neurotic symptoms, depression, separation-anxiety, self-esteem, body-image. Overprotection and favouring by parents. Recalcitrance. Expectancies/ideals for the future.
Intellectual variables:	IQ (intelligence quotient).
Social variables:	Schoolfunctioning and -achievements. Leisure-time activities. Social competence and -inhibitions. Problems with insurances, medical examinations and financial costs related to CHD. Rejection for the Army. Choice of profession, difficulties in getting a job, employment status. Sexual relations, marital status and pregnancies.

Statistical analyses will be carried out for the sample as a whole and will be differentiated for the five separate diagnostic groups. In the near future we intend to publish the results of this study.

Acknowledgements

This study was financially supported by a research grant from the Netherlands Heart Foundation (JH 8802).

References

1. Maxwell GM, Gane S. The impact of congenital heart disease upon the family. Am Heart J 1962;64(4):449–54.
2. Glaser HH, Harrison GS, Lynn DB. Emotional implications of congenital heart disease in children. Pediatrics 1964; March:367–79.
3. Garson A, Benson RS, Ivler L, Patton C. Parental reactions to children with congenital heart disease. Child Psych Human Dev 1978;9:86–94.
4. Donovan E. The pediatric cardiologist and adolescents with congenital heart disease. Int J Cardiol 1983;9:493–5.
5. Sutherland GR, Hess J, Roelandt J, Quaegebeur J. Editorial. The increasing problem of young adults with congenital heart disease. Eur Heart J 1990;11:4–6.

6. Garson SL, Baer PE. Psychological aspects of heart disease in childhood. In: Garson JR A, Bricker JT, McNamara DG, editors. The science and practice of pediatric cardiology. Philadelphia/London: Lea & Febiger, 1990:2519–27.

7. Linde LM, Adams FH, Rozansky GI. Physical and emotional aspects of congenital heart disease in children. Am J Cardiol 1971;27:712–3.

8. Linde LM. Psychiatric aspects of congenital heart disease. Psych Clin North Am 1982;5(2):399–406.

9. Varnauskas E, de Fernández YL, Muñoz S, Williams WH, Hatcher CR, James FW. Rehabilitation of pediatric and adolescent cardiac patients. In: Wenger NK, Almeida-Feo D, Rosenthal J, editors. Advances in cardiology (Vol. 33). Basel: Karger, 1986:131–41.

10. Bowen J. Helping children and their families cope with congenital heart disease. Crit Care Q 1985;8(3):65–74.

11. Offord DR, Cross LA, Andrews EJ, Aponte JF. Perceived and actual severity of congenital heart disease and effect on family life. Psychosomatics 1972;13(6):390–6.

12. Kitchen LW. Psychological factors in congenital heart disease in children. J Fam Pract 1978;6(4):390–6.

13. Brodie B. Views of healthy children towards illness. Am J Public Health 1974;64(12):1158.

14. Fowler MG, Johnson MP, Welshimer KJ, Atkinson SS, Loda FA. Factors related to school absence among children with cardiac conditions. Am J Dis Child 1987;141(12):1317–20.

15. O'Dougherty M, Wright FS, Garmezy N, Loewenson RB, Torres F. Later competence and adaptation in infants who survive severe heart defects. Child Dev 1983;54:1129–42.

16. Newburger JW, Sibert AR, Buckley LP, Fyler DC. Cognitive function and age at repair of transposition of the great arteries in children. N Eng J Med 1984;310(23):1495–9.

17. Thomas-Van Moerbeke RM, Debaise I, Vliers A. Enfants cardiaques opérés sous hypothermie profonde dans les premiers mois. Arch Fr Pediatr 1986;43:691–4.

18. Wells FC, Coghill S, Caplan HL, Lincoln C. Duration of circulatory arrest does influence the psychological development of children after cardiac operation in early life. J Thorac Cardiovasc Surg 1983;86:823–31.

19. Silverman S. Family adaptation to congenital heart disease: adjusting to physical and moral realities. In: Anderson RH et al., editors. Pediatric Cardiology, Vol 5. New York: Churchill Livingstone 1983:317–26.

20. Ghisla R, Stocker F, Weber JW, Schüpbach P. Psychosoziale Auswirkungen des Herzfehlers im Adoleszenten- und Erwachsenenalter bei Tertalogie von Fallot. Schweiz Med Wochenschr, 1983;113:20–4.

21. Gabriel HP, Danilowicz D. Postoperative responses in 'prepared' child after cardiac surgery. Br Heart J 1978;40:1046–51.

22. Wright, M, Jarvis S, Wannamaker E, Cook D. Congenital heart disease: Functional abilities in young adults. Arch Phys Med Rehabil 1985;66:289–93.

23. Otterstad JE, Tjore I, Sundby P. Social function of adults with isolated ventricular septal defects. Scand J Soc Med 1986;4:15–23.

24. Jedlicka-Köhler I, Wimmer M. Der Einfluss des Operationszeitpunktes auf die intellektuelle und Psychosoziale Entwicklung bei Kindern mit Fallotscher Tetralogie. Klin Paediatrie 1987;199:86–9.

25. Baer PE, Freedman DA, Garson A. Long-term psychological follow-up of patients after corrective surgery for Tetralogy of Fallot. J Am Acad Child Psychiatry 1984;23(5):662–5.

Index

Developments in Cardiovascular Medicine

50. J. Meyer, R. Erbel and H.J. Rupprecht (eds.): *Improvement of Myocardial Perfusion*. Thrombolysis, Angioplasty, Bypass Surgery. Proceedings of a Symposium, held in Mainz, F.R.G. (1984). 1985   ISBN 0-89838-748-5
51. J.H.C. Reiber, P.W. Serruys and C.J. Slager (eds.): *Quantitative Coronary and Left Ventricular Cineangiography*. Methodology and Clinical Applications. 1986
                                                                          ISBN 0-89838-760-4
52. R.H. Fagard and I.E. Bekaert (eds.): *Sports Cardiology*. Exercise in Health and Cardiovascular Disease. Proceedings from an International Conference, held in Knokke, Belgium (1985). 1986   ISBN 0-89838-782-5
53. J.H.C. Reiber and P.W. Serruys (eds.): *State of the Art in Quantitative Cornary Arteriography*. 1986   ISBN 0-89838-804-X
54. J. Roelandt (ed.): *Color Doppler Flow Imaging and Other Advances in Doppler Echocardiography*. 1986   ISBN 0-89838-806-6
55. E.E. van der Wall (ed.): *Noninvasive Imaging of Cardiac Metabolism*. Single Photon Scintigraphy, Positron Emission Tomography and Nuclear Magnetic Resonance. 1987
                                                                          ISBN 0-89838-812-0
56. J. Liebman, R. Plonsey and Y. Rudy (eds.): *Pediatric and Fundamental Electrocardiography*. 1987   ISBN 0-89838-815-5
57. H.H. Hilger, V. Hombach and W.J. Rashkind (eds.), *Invasive Cardiovascular Therapy*. Proceedings of an International Symposium, held in Cologne, F.R.G. (1985). 1987   ISBN 0-89838-818-X
58. P.W. Serruys and G.T. Meester (eds.): *Coronary Angioplasty*. A Controlled Model for Ischemia. 1986   ISBN 0-89838-819-8
59. J.E. Tooke and L.H. Smaje (eds.): *Clinical Investigation of the Microcirculation*. Proceedings of an International Meeting, held in London, U.K. (1985). 1987
                                                                          ISBN 0-89838-833-3
60. R.Th. van Dam and A. van Oosterom (eds.): *Electrocardiographic Body Surface Mapping*. Proceedings of the 3rd International Symposium on B.S.M., held in Nijmegen, The Netherlands (1985). 1986   ISBN 0-89838-834-1
61. M.P. Spencer (ed.): *Ultrasonic Diagnosis of Cerebrovascular Disease*. Doppler Techniques and Pulse Echo Imaging. 1987   ISBN 0-89838-836-8
62. M.J. Legato (ed.): *The Stressed Heart*. 1987   ISBN 0-89838-849-X
63. M.E. Safar (ed.): *Arterial and Venous Systems in Essential Hypertension*. With Assistance of G.M. London, A.Ch. Simon and Y.A. Weiss. 1987
                                                                          ISBN 0-89838-857-0
64. J. Roelandt (ed.): *Digital Techniques in Echocardiography*. 1987
                                                                          ISBN 0-89838-861-9
65. N.S. Dhalla, P.K. Singal and R.E. Beamish (eds.): *Pathology of Heart Disease*. Proceedings of the 8th Annual Meeting of the American Section of the I.S.H.R., held in Winnipeg, Canada, 1986 (Vol. 1). 1987   ISBN 0-89838-864-3
66. N.S. Dhalla, G.N. Pierce and R.E. Beamish (eds.): *Heart Function and Metabolism*. Proceedings of the 8th Annual Meeting of the American Section of the I.S.H.R., held in Winnipeg, Canada, 1986 (Vol. 2). 1987   ISBN 0-89838-865-1
67. N.S. Dhalla, I.R. Innes and R.E. Beamish (eds.): *Myocardial Ischemia*. Proceedings of a Satellite Symposium of the 30th International Physiological Congress, held in Winnipeg, Canada (1986). 1987   ISBN 0-89838-866-X
68. R.E. Beamish, V. Panagia and N.S. Dhalla (eds.): *Pharmacological Aspects of Heart Disease*. Proceedings of an International Symposium, held in Winnipeg, Canada (1986). 1987   ISBN 0-89838-867-8
69. H.E.D.J. ter Keurs and J.V. Tyberg (eds.): *Mechanics of the Circulation*. Proceedings of a Satellite Symposium of the 30th International Physiological Congress, held in Banff, Alberta, Canada (1986). 1987   ISBN 0-89838-870-8
70. S. Sideman and R. Beyar (eds.): *Activation, Metabolism and Perfusion of the Heart*. Simulation and Experimental Models. Proceedings of the 3rd Henry Goldberg Workshop, held in Piscataway, N.J., U.S.A. (1986). 1987   ISBN 0-89838-871-6

Developments in Cardiovascular Medicine

Developments in Cardiovascular Medicine

96. I. Cikes (ed.): *Echocardiography in Cardiac Interventions.* 1989
ISBN 0-7923-0088-2
97. E. Rapaport (ed.): *Early Interventions in Acute Myocardial Infarction.* 1989
ISBN 0-7923-0175-7
98. M.E. Safar and F. Fouad-Tarazi (eds.): *The Heart in Hypertension.* A Tribute to Robert C. Tarazi (1925-1986). 1989 ISBN 0-7923-0197-8
99. S. Meerbaum and R. Meltzer (eds.): *Myocardial Contrast Two-dimensional Echocardiography.* 1989 ISBN 0-7923-0205-2
100. J. Morganroth and E.N. Moore (eds.): *Risk/Benefit Analysis for the Use and Approval of Thrombolytic, Antiarrhythmic, and Hypolipidemic Agents.* Proceedings of the 9th Annual Symposium on New Drugs and Devices (1988). 1989 ISBN 0-7923-0294-X
101. P.W. Serruys, R. Simon and K.J. Beatt (eds.): *PTCA - An Investigational Tool and a Non-operative Treatment of Acute Ischemia.* 1990 ISBN 0-7923-0346-6
102. I.S. Anand, P.I. Wahi and N.S. Dhalla (eds.): *Pathophysiology and Pharmacology of Heart Disease.* 1989 ISBN 0-7923-0367-9
103. G.S. Abela (ed.): *Lasers in Cardiovascular Medicine and Surgery.* Fundamentals and Technique. 1990 ISBN 0-7923-0440-3
104. H.M. Piper (ed.): *Pathophysiology of Severe Ischemic Myocardial Injury.* 1990
ISBN 0-7923-0459-4
105. S.M. Teague (ed.): *Stress Doppler Echocardiography.* 1990 ISBN 0-7923-0499-3
106. P.R. Saxena, D.I. Wallis, W. Wouters and P. Bevan (eds.): *Cardiovascular Pharmacology of 5-Hydroxytryptamine.* Prospective Therapeutic Applications. 1990
ISBN 0-7923-0502-7
107. A.P. Shepherd and P.A. Öberg (eds.): *Laser-Doppler Blood Flowmetry.* 1990
ISBN 0-7923-0508-6
108. J. Soler-Soler, G. Permanyer-Miralda and J. Sagristà-Sauleda (eds.): *Pericardial Disease.* New Insights and Old Dilemmas. 1990 ISBN 0-7923-0510-8
109. J.P.M. Hamer: *Practical Echocardiography in the Adult.* With Doppler and Color-Doppler Flow Imaging. 1990 ISBN 0-7923-0670-8
110. A. Bayés de Luna, P. Brugada, J. Cosin Aguilar and F. Navarro Lopez (eds.): *Sudden Cardiac Death.* 1991 ISBN 0-7923-0716-X
111. E. Andries and R. Stroobandt (eds.): *Hemodynamics in Daily Practice.* 1991
ISBN 0-7923-0725-9
112. J. Morganroth and E.N. Moore (eds.): *Use and Approval of Antihypertensive Agents and Surrogate Endpoints for the Approval of Drugs affecting Antiarrhythmic Heart Failure and Hypolipidemia.* Proceedings of the 10th Annual Symposium on New Drugs and Devices (1989). 1990 ISBN 0-7923-0756-9
113. S. Iliceto, P. Rizzon and J.R.T.C. Roelandt (eds.): *Ultrasound in Coronary Artery Disease.* Present Role and Future Perspectives. 1990 ISBN 0-7923-0784-4
114. J.V. Chapman and G.R. Sutherland (eds.): *The Noninvasive Evaluation of Hemodynamics in Congenital Heart Disease.* Doppler Ultrasound Applications in the Adult and Pediatric Patient with Congenital Heart Disease. 1990
ISBN 0-7923-0836-0
115. G.T. Meester and F. Pinciroli (eds.): *Databases for Cardiology.* 1991
ISBN 0-7923-0886-7
116. B. Korecky and N.S. Dhalla (eds.): *Subcellular Basis of Contractile Failure.* 1990
ISBN 0-7923-0890-5
117. J.H.C. Reiber and P.W. Serruys (eds.): *Quantitative Coronary Arteriography.* 1991
ISBN 0-7923-0913-8
118. E. van der Wall and A. de Roos (eds.): *Magnetic Resonance Imaging in Coronary Artery Disease.* 1991 ISBN 0-7923-0940-5
119. V. Hombach, M. Kochs and A.J. Camm (eds.): *Interventional Techniques in Cardiovascular Medicine.* 1991 ISBN 0-7923-0956-1
120. R. Vos: *Drugs Looking for Diseases.* Innovative Drug Research and the Development of the Beta Blockers and the Calcium Antagonists. 1991 ISBN 0-7923-0968-5

Developments in Cardiovascular Medicine

Previous volumes are still available

KLUWER ACADEMIC PUBLISHERS – DORDRECHT / BOSTON / LONDON